PIGS:

The Homoeopathic Approach
to the Treatment and
Prevention of

PIGS:

The Homoeopathic Approach to the Treatment and Prevention of Diseases

by
GEORGE MACLEOD
MRCVS, DVSM, Vet. FF Hom

Veterinary Fellow of the Faculty of Homoeopathy

Index compiled by Lyn Greenwood

SAFFRON WALDEN
THE C.W. DANIEL COMPANY LIMITED

First published in Great Britain by
The C.W. Daniel Company Limited
1 Church Path, Saffron Walden
Essex, CB10 1JP, England

ISBN 978 0 85207 278 3

4

Penguin Random House is committed to a sustainable future for
our business, our readers and our planet. This book is made from
Forest Stewardship Council® certified paper.

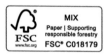

Printed and bound in Great Britain by Clays Ltd, St Ives plc

Production in association with
Book Production Consultants Plc, Cambridge
Typeset by Cambridge Photosetting

CONTENTS

PREFACE

THIS OUTLINE of the commoner pig diseases has been written in response to a growing demand on the part of pig farmers for a producer's text-book which will provide a working manual to which reference can readily be made. No claim is made that it is exhaustive or complete in every detail and many remedies not listed may be needed depending on particular symptoms in any one condition. However the main ones have been listed. The potencies of remedies are a guide only and here again different ones may be needed. A good general guide is to use low potencies, e.g. 6c for the treatment of chronic conditions while reserving the higher potencies for those showing more acute symptoms. Repetition of the remedy is also a matter which will depend greatly on the response and progress of any condition. Acute affections may need three or four doses in twenty-four hours, while less acute ones could have the frequency reduced to twice weekly. Much will depend on the individual case and in this connection professional advice is always available.

I am grateful to Mosby-Year Book Europe for permission to refer to the publication "Diseases of Swine" – 7th Edition (Leman and others).

Finally I would like to thank my secretary Mrs. Enid Abbott for giving up some of her leisure time to typing the manuscript and for persevering in the face of some rather unusual nomenclature.

INTRODUCTION

*T*HE TREATMENT of pigs by homoeopathy presents diffi-
culties which do not arise when the same form of treatment
is carried out in other species. This is because oral administration is particularly difficult in older animals, although this
method is relatively easy in piglets and other young animals.

As the great majority of pig diseases are specific in nature
(i.e. bacterial or viral orientated) it was decided to omit a
general description of non-specific conditions affecting the
various body systems as is the case in other publications by
the author relating to other species.

The exceptions to this are the chapters dealing with
affections of the skin, reproductive and urogenital systems.

We would emphasise the importance of the prophylactic
approach to disease control of pig diseases by homoeopathic
means. This relies on the use of nosodes against the various
conditions (see chapter on nosodes).

Although the following pages concentrate on the treatment and prevention of disease it must be emphasised that
management and proper housing are of paramount importance in maintaining an environment which is favourable
to the employment of the remedies. In other words any
system which produces stress and overcrowding together
with inadequate ventilation will inevitably reduce the efficacy
of the remedies. It is essential therefore that management
practices will take this into account.

Not all of the diseases discussed in the text are of interest to pig producers in the United Kingdom but they have been included in the hope that they may be of interest to pig farmers in other countries. Also some of the diseases discussed are subject to restrictions under the Diseases of Animals Acts and Orders, but they have been included in the hope that owners may recognise the cardinal symptoms of these diseases and take action accordingly.

The nature of Homoeopathic Remedies

Homoeopathic remedies are obtained from all natural sources, e.g. the plant and animal kingdoms and also minerals and their compounds. Homoeopathy is frequently referred to – quite erroneously – as herbal medicine. Nothing could be further from the truth as consideration of the above remarks will show. While herbal medicine employs many plants successfully it is unable to exploit the intrinsic merits of plants in the way that homoeopathic medicine is able to do.

Preparation of Remedies

Preparation of homoeopathic remedies is a scientific procedure which is best left to a qualified pharmacist trained in the essential techniques. Homoeopathy is too important for remedies to be prepared in any way but the best obtainable.

Briefly the system is based on a series of dilutions and succussions (see below) which is capable of rendering even a poisonous substance safe to use.

To prepare a potentised remedy, a measured drop of a solution called mother tincture – expressed as the Greek letter ø – derived from plant or other material is added to 99 drops of a water/alcohol mixture in a test tube. The resultant solution is subjected to a mechanical shock which is called succussion. This process which is essential to the preparation imparts energy to the medium which is then rendered stable. One drop of ø to 99 parts of water/alcohol mixture is represented by 1c on the centesimal scale. Preparations are also made on the decimal scale (one drop to 10 parts alcohol/water). These are marketed as 1x (on the continent as D). Repeated dilutions and succussions yield higher potencies releasing more energy in the process. It will be appreciated therefore that homoeopathy is a system of medicine which concerns itself with energy and not with material doses of a drug.

Selection of Potencies

Once the simillimum or 'most likely' remedy has been selected the question of which potency to use arises. As a general rule in the author's experience the higher potencies (1m–10m) which are more energised than the lower should be employed in acute infections while the lower (6c–30c) should be reserved for chronic conditions with or without pathological changes being present. It will be found occasionally that there are exceptions to this point of view and indeed many practitioners especially on the continent rely mostly on lower potencies for general use.

The potencies mentioned under each remedy in the text are a guide only. Higher potencies will necessitate professional advice.

Administration of Remedies

Remedies are marketed as medicated tablets and powders and also as tinctures and water dilutions. When treating piglets and weaners it should be relatively easy to treat the individual animal orally by emptying the remedy (preferably in powder form) directly on to the animal's tongue when the essence of the remedy will quickly be absorbed into the system. The treatment of large animals necessitates a different approach and in this case the remedy should be given in drinking water. This also applies to the prophylactic use of nosodes (see below).

Care of Remedies

The delicate nature of homoeopathic remedies which is inherent in their preparation renders them subject to contamination by strong-smelling substances, e.g. camphor, scents, disinfectants, etc. and also by strong sunlight. It is essential therefore that they be kept away from such influences and stored in a cool dry place out of strong sunlight. The use of amber glass bottles is helpful in this connection for the storage of tablets.

Nosodes and Oral Vaccines

It will be noticed in the text under treatment of various specific conditions that reference is made to the term 'nosode', and it is necessary to explain fully to what the term refers. A nosode (from the Greek NOSOS, meaning disease) is a disease product obtained from any part of the system in a case of illness and thereafter potentised in the same way as for ordinary remedies, e.g. respiratory secretions from a case of Pasteurella Pneumonia or bowel secretions from a case of Swine Dysentery. In specific (bacterial, viral and protozoal disease) the causative organism may or may not be present in the material and the efficacy of the nosode in no way depends on the organism being present. The response of the tissues to invasion by bacteria or viruses results in the formation of substances which are in effect the basis of the nosode.

Oral vaccines are prepared from the actual organism

which causes a disease and may derive from filtrates containing only the exotoxins of the bacteria, or from emulsions containing both bacteria and their toxins. These filtrates and emulsions are then potentised and become oral vaccines.

There are two ways of employing nosodes and oral vaccines:

1. THERAPEUTICALLY AND 2. PROPHYLACTICALLY

When we employ nosodes therapeutically we may use them for the condition from which the nosode was derived, e.g. Swine Dysentery in the treatment of that disease. This may be termed isopathic (treatment with a substance from an animal suffering from the *same* disease): or we may employ the nosode in any condition the symptoms of which resemble the symptom-complex of the particular nosode, e.g. the use of the nosode *PSORINUM* in the treatment of the particular form of skin disease which appears in the provings of that nosode. This may be termed homoeopathic (treatment with a substance taken from an animal suffering from a *similar* disease). In this connection it must be remembered that many nosodes have been proved in their own right (each has its own particular drug picture). Many veterinary nosodes have been developed but no provings exist for them and they are used almost entirely in the treatment or prevention of the associated diseases.

AUTONOSODES

This particular type of nosode is prepared from material provided by the individual patient, e.g. pus from a chronic sinus or fistula and after potentisation used for the treatment of the same patient. Autonosodes are usually employed in refractory cases where well-indicated remedies have failed to produce the desired results and frequently they produce striking results.

ORAL VACCINES

As with nosodes oral vaccines may be used both thera-peutically and prophylactically. If the condition is caused wholly by bacterial or viral invasion the use of the oral vaccine is frequently attended by spectacular results, but this is less likely when there is an underlying chronic condition complicating an acute infection. Here we may need the help of constitutional and/or other remedies.

BOWEL NOSODES

The bowel nosodes comprise a special group derived from the non-lactose fermenting bacteria of the bowel, viz. the *Salmonella* and *E. coli* families. Research on this subject by the late Dr. John Paterson showed that an increase in the number of such organisms followed treatment by particular homoeopathic remedies. He therefore concluded that these particular nosodes were associated with particular remedies.

The bowel nosodes which concern us in veterinary practice are as follows:

1. MORGAN 2. PROTEUS 3. GAERTNER 4. DYS CO 5. SYCOTIC CO

MORGAN Clinical observations have revealed the symp-tom-picture of the bacillus Morgan to cover in general digestive and respiratory systems with an action also on fibrous tissue and skin. It is used principally in the treatment of inflammatory skin conditions combined with an associated remedy, these being one of *SULPHUR, GRAPHITES, PETROLEUM* and *PSORINUM*.

PROTEUS The central and peripheral nervous systems figure prominently in the clinical picture of this nosode, e.g. convulsions and seizures together with spasm of the peripheral circulation; cramping of muscles is a common feature; angio-neurotic oedema frequently occurs and there is a marked sensitivity to ultra-violet light. Associated remedies are *CUPRUM METALLICUM* and *NATRUM MURIATICUM.*

GAERTNER Marked emaciation and/or malnutrition is associated with this nosode. Chronic gastroenteritis occurs and there is a tendency for the animal to become infested with worms. There is an inability to digest fat. Associated remedies are *MERC CORR, PHOSPHORUS* and *SILICEA.*

DYS CO. This nosode is chiefly concerned with disturbances of the digestive and cardiac systems. Pyloric spasm occurs with retention of digested stomach contents leading to vomiting. There is functional disturbance of the heart's action, usually as a result of tension. Associated remedies are *ARSENICUM ALBUM, ARGENTUM NITRICUM* and *KALMIA LATIFOLIA.*

SYCOTIC CO. The keynote of this nosode is sub-acute or chronic inflammation of mucous membranes especially those of the intestinal tract where a chronic catarrhal enteritis develops. Chronic bronchitis and nasal catarrh have also been noted. Associated remedies are *MERC CORR, NITRIC ACID* and *HYDRASTIS.*

MAIN INDICATIONS FOR THE USE OF BOWEL NOSODES

When a case is presented showing one or two leading symptoms which suggest a particular remedy we should employ that remedy, if necessary in varying potencies, before abandoning it and resorting to another if unsatisfactory results ensue. In chronic disease there may be conflicting symptoms which suggest several competing remedies and it is here that the bowel nosodes may be used with advantage. A study of the associated remedies will usually lead us to the particular nosode to be employed. The question of potency and repetition of dosage assumes special importance when considering the use of bowel nosodes. The low to medium potencies, e.g. 6c–30c are more suitable for this purpose than the higher ones and can be safely administered daily for a few days. Bowel nosodes are deep-acting remedies and should not be repeated until a few months have elapsed since the previous prescription.

I am indebted to the late Dr John Paterson for his observations on and research into the bowel nosodes.

Vaccination procedure

This is based on the use of nosodes and/or oral vaccines. There is no hard and fast rule concerning frequency of administration but a system which has yielded satisfactory results is to give a single dose – preferably in powder form – night and morning for three days, followed by one per week for four weeks. This is the procedure which should be followed for piglets up to weaning stage. Where young pigs are to be kept for breeding this regime can be extended to cover a further dose monthly for six months.

In the case of adult animals – sows, gilts and boars – vaccination should be carried out via the drinking water. A suggested course of action which has proved satisfactory is first to dissolve ten powders in 500ml of distilled water, preferably in an amber glass bottle. From this stock solution 10ml can be added to the drinking water per week for eight weeks. After an interval of two weeks this procedure can be repeated. This should build up an adequate resistance to most of the commoner infections.

There is a fundamental difference between conventional vaccination and that using the oral route. The former involves the subcutaneous or intramuscular injection of an antigen (vaccine material) which after an interval of ten or twenty days produces antibodies in the blood stream against the particular antigen – described usually as humoral antibody response. While in most cases by this method a degree of protection against the particular disease is established, the procedure can be criticised on two grounds:

1. The defence system is not fully incorporated by this means and
2. there is a risk of side-effects due to the foreign nature of the protein factor involved in the vaccine. This aspect of conventional vaccination has been well documented in other species.

By contrast oral vaccination gives a more solid immunity inasmuch as it incorporates the entire defence system which is mobilised as soon as the vaccine is taken into the mouth and builds up protection with each further dose. This build-up leads on from tonsillar tissue through the lymphatics finally engaging the entire reticulo-endothelial system. This procedure is equivalent to what is known as "street infection" viz. ingestion of virus etc. during daily contact with animals which are already infected or shedding virus from time to time. Another advantage to protection by homoeopathic means is that piglets can be treated in the first week of life if necessary which removes the necessity of waiting until maternal antibodies have been eliminated from the system, as nosodes can produce their protection even in the presence of these antibodies.

VACCINATION FAILURE

Even though they have been vaccinated some animals may develop disease and this could occur on account of various factors e.g. incubation of disease may be taking place at the time the vaccine is administered. Again contamination of the vaccine may be a factor. Occasionally also immuno-suppression may be a factor preventing successful vaccination.

CHAPTER ONE

DISEASES
of the Skin

MANY OF THESE conditions will be dealt with under specific diseases (q.v.) but other more simple conditions can be considered:

1. ABSCESSES. These are occasionally encountered and are associated with various strains of bacteria, e.g. *Streptococci* and *Actinomyces* particularly. These abscesses are identified as swellings beneath the skin, the skin above appearing as a reddish discolouration. Areas around the flank, ears and shoulders are the commonest sites of infection. Streptococcal infection is also involved in the production of abscesses in the glands below the jaw. Specific infections can lead to septicaemia in young piglets, the skin showing small haemorrhages in the region of the abdomen and flank. Older animals, especially sows, develop abscesses along the flanks and on the back and neck.

2. A specific form of skin disease is associated with infection by the organism Staphyloccocus Hyius causing an exudative condition of the skin known as *Exudative Epidermitis* – also known in some quarters as Greasy Pig Disease. It mostly affects young pigs between one and eight weeks of age. Acute forms of this condition present as secretions from sebaceous glands which show as smelly greasy lesions, commencing on the facial areas and extending to the majority of the skin surfaces.

➤ **TREATMENT**
Abscesses usually respond to treatment utilising remedies such as Hepar Sulph and/or Silicea. Acute abscesses which are tender to the touch are treatable by Hepar Sulph in differing potencies dependent on the stage of abscess development. Early abscess formation where there is sensitivity to touch should be treated with high (1m–10m) potencies while lower potencies (6c–12c) should be employed to promote rapid maturation of the abscess and to hasten the healing process. The main remedies to consider in the treatment of Exudative Dermatitis are *SULPHUR* 30c one dose daily for ten days, followed by *GRAPHITES* 1m three times per week for four weeks. Other remedies to consider if these prove unsatisfactory are *PSORINUM* 30c and *MEZEREUM* 30c.

*C*ontagious *Pyoderma*
This condition affecting young piglets occasionally occurs. It also affects the mammary glands of sows from which spread to piglets may take place. It is associated with strains of Streptococci.

➤ **CLINICAL SIGNS**
A rise in temperature is followed by an appearance of depression and reddening of the skin. The abdominal area may show superficial haemorrhages while pustules develop in various body areas e.g. inguinal and around facial structures. Pustules are followed by scab formation as in pox lesions.

> **TREATMENT**

1. GUNPOWDER. This remedy has a well-proven record in the treatment of pustular conditions as described. A potency of 6c should be used giving it three times per day for seven days.

2. HEPAR SULPH. A potency of 30c should be helpful in most cases giving it once daily for fourteen days.

3. VARIOLINUM. Although the condition is unrelated to the pox diseases the symptom picture suggests that this nosode could be effective in some cases. A potency of 30c should be given daily for ten days.

4. ECHINACEA. Symptoms associated with a rise in temperature accompanying multiple small papules/pustules in various parts of the body may be alleviated by this remedy. It is best employed in low potencies, e.g. 6c three times daily for ten days.

5. STREPTOCOCCUS NOSODE. A combined Streptococcus nosode should also be helpful, e.g. Streptococcus 30c giving a daily dose for seven days along with selected remedies.

*F*ungal *Skin Disease*

The fungus *Candida albicans* is capable of causing a dermatitis manifested as circular lesions on the abdominal area and hind limbs. These lesions may exude a greyish moist material. The skin becomes thickened and hairless and may assume a bluish colour.

> **TREATMENT**

1. SULPHUR. This is usually indicated as a preliminary remedy and may be combined with the remedy *MORGAN*. The skin surrounding the lesion is often warm to the touch.

Suggested potencies for *SULPHUR* range from 30c to 200c. *MORGAN* should be given in 30c daily for five days and followed by *SULPHUR* 30c once daily for seven days. If potencies of 200c seem indicated once per week for four weeks should suffice.

2. GRAPHITES. The moist exudate which accompanies the lesions should respond to treatment with this remedy. Suggested potency 30c daily for ten days.

3. HEPAR SULPH. This remedy should suffice to ward off secondary infection involving any lesion. It will also relieve pain and sensitivity of the skin. A potency of 30c should be given daily for seven days.

4. LACHESIS. If the lesions on the abdominal and inguinal areas are accompanied by bluish–purple discolouration to any significant degree this remedy may be indicated and should give satisfactory results. Suggested potency 30c once daily for seven days.

5. ARSEN ALB. This remedy should be of benefit in the treatment of thickened skin and will promote growth of hair. Suggested potency 1m daily for ten days.

6. CANDIDA ALBICANS 30C. This nosode given in 30c potency daily for seven days should accompany any selected remedy.

*R*ingworm

Porcine ringworm is caused by fungal agents called *Microsporum* and *Trichophyton* (various types of each). Once infection establishes itself in a herd, spread can take place extensively affecting pigs of all ages.

➤ CLINICAL SIGNS

Reddish circular lesions appear on various parts of the body ultimately progressing into dry scabby areas: the abdominal area is usually unaffected. Contrary to the condition affecting other species itching is unusual. The condition is important because of the possibility of spread to those handling pigs or otherwise coming into contact with them.

➤ TREATMENT

1. BACILLINUM. This nosode has a proven record in the treatment of ringworm in various species. It should be prescribed in 200c one dose per week for six weeks.

2. SEPIA. The typical lesions resemble those which appear in the provings of the remedy and can be used in conjunction with the above remedy or by itself in milder outbreaks. Suggested potency 200c once per week for four weeks.

3. MICROSPORUM AND TRICHOPHYTON NOSODES. Compound nosodes in 30c potency should accompany selected remedies giving a dose daily for seven days.

Sunburn and Photosensitization

Pigs grazing outside in prolonged sunny weather may be affected with either or both of these conditions. Sunburn produces excessive heat and redness together with oedema especially behind the ears. Pain associated with the condition may affect the gait of the affected animal. In severe cases the skin may eventually peel off. Photosensitization also occurs under similar circumstances but in this condition there is a triggering factor associated with the ingestion of various plants or grasses, e.g. St. Johns Wort, rape and alfalfa. Another point of difference is that it affects only

5

white breeds, pigmented areas remaining unaffected. As in sunburn the skin becomes hot and oedematous and eventually peels off leaving a raw surface which is extremely itchy.

➤ **TREATMENT**

1. SUNBURN. The main remedy to consider is *BELLADONNA* which will relieve the heat in the skin and prevent progression deepening. A potency of 200c should suffice giving one dose daily for seven days. The remedy *APIS MEL* will be helpful in controlling the oedema which develops.

2. PHOTOSENSITIZATION. Belladonna will also prove useful as above, but it should be combined with *HYPERICUM* lm daily for seven or ten days. Raw areas appearing after sloughing of skin should be bathed with *HYPERCAL* lotion diluted 1/10 with warm water. (Hypercal is a combination of the remedies Calendula and Hypericum prepared for external use.)

*H*aematoma

This term denotes any fluctuating swelling appearing on any part of the body as a result of bruising which causes extravasation of blood which collects in localised pockets. The commonest site of this condition is the ear flap resulting from repeated shaking of the head due to different types of otitis. These swellings usually resolve themselves gradually once the fluid part of the blood is resorbed. The remedy *ARNICA* is the main remedy to consider and will hasten the healing process considerably. It should be given in 30c potency once daily for ten days.

Pityriasis Rosea or Pustular Psoriaform Dermatitis

This is a condition of unknown etiology which can affect young pigs especially those of the Landrace breed and manifests as reddish papules which are hot to the touch and concentrate on the abdomen and inguinal areas. These lesions tend to spread and coalesce into different shapes. Occasionally the lesions affect the dorsum but are less severe in this area.

➤ TREATMENT

1. SULPHUR. This remedy in 30c along with MORGAN 30c should be given as early as possible. A daily dose of each for seven days should suffice.

2. MEZEREUM. This is a remedy which has given good results in this and similar cases in other species particularly when back lesions predominate. A potency of 200c daily for seven days is indicated.

3. PETROLEUM. This remedy should also be considered especially in those cases accompanied by fissures surrounding the periphery of the lesions. Suggested potency 30c twice daily for ten days.

There is a theory that the condition may be hereditary.

Dermatosis Vegetans

This is considered to be hereditary and appears early in the piglet's life.

➤ CLINICAL SIGNS

The piglets develop swelling and heat around the coronary structure particularly of the front feet (although hind feet

7

can show lesions also). A yellowish exudate develops on the skin above the feet. Lesions of dermatitis taking the form of small papules develop on the abdomen and inguinal area. These papules tend to coalesce forming raised areas covered by scaly material. The horn of the hoof becomes affected forming ridges and furrows running horizontally. Systemic involvement is manifested by increased respiration and altered expiration.

➤ TREATMENT

1. HEPAR SULPH. This remedy should help in the early stages limiting the development of swelling and relieving pain etc. Suggested potency 30c twice daily for seven days.

2. VARIOLINUM. This nosode will help limit the spread of papular lesions and help them resolve quickly. Suggested potency 200c once daily for seven days.

3. PHOSPHORUS. Respiratory involvement may be relieved by this remedy in a potency of 200c giving it once daily for five days. It is just one of many competing remedies in this connection, others being *AMMON CARB, SULPHUROUS ACID* and *AMYL NITRITE* all in 30c potency.

4. SILICEA. Lesions around the coronary band will benefit from this remedy. It will also have a beneficial action on the hoof wall producing hardening and removing ridges and furrows.

*H*yperkeratinisation

This is a condition characterised by the development of dark greasy scales on the back and behind the ears and affecting adult housed animals. It is considered to be dietary in origin.

➤ TREATMENT

MORGAN 30c and *SULPHUR* 30c should be employed first once daily each for seven days. *GRAPHITES* 30c should follow these giving one dose daily for ten days. Normally these remedies should suffice but others which may be indicated depending on overall symptoms are *ARSEN ALB* and *IODUM*.

CHAPTER TWO

AFFECTIONS
of the Urinary Tract

URINARY TRACT INFECTION could be dependent on systemic bacterial or viral diseases especially those associated with *Streptococci* and *Salmonella* organisms. Local infections of the urinary tract arise from ascending infection from bladder or urethra when frequent urination develops, the urine itself containing purulent material containing strains of *E. coli*.

Cystitis and Pyelonephritis

These conditions are usually studied together in the pig and are seldom if ever seen in young animals, sows and boars being pre-eminently affected. Ascending infection via the urethra is primarily responsible for the development of these conditions and can cause death in severe cases.

➤ ETIOLOGY

Specific bacteria of the *E. coli*, *Klebsiella* and *Streptococcus* families are primarily responsible, although *Corynebacteria* have recently been found to play a major part.

➤ CLINICAL SIGNS

Blood in urine accompanied by purulent staining around the genital area are early signs. Severe cases exhibit systemic signs such as frequent urination, excessive thirst and increased blood in urine. Loss of condition is commonplace.

➤ **TREATMENT**

1. BERBERIS VULGARIS. Early haematuria (blood in urine) should respond to this remedy employing a potency of 30c twice daily for seven days.

2. HEPAR SULPH. This is one of the main remedies used in homoeopathic medicine to combat infections which are purulent in nature. Given in high potency in this condition, e.g. 1m it will limit the spread of the disease and help localise it.

3. E. COLI and **CORYNEBACTERIUM** nosodes are also indicated giving them daily in 30c potency along with other remedies.

4. ECHINACEA. Systemic involvement may need this remedy as it has proved useful in septicaemic disturbances given in low potency, e.g. 6c three times daily for five days.

CHAPTER THREE

MUSCULO-*skeletal system*

LAMENESS DEPENDENT ON abnormalities or disease of bones can be a major cause of economic loss in pig units more especially if it affects a significant number of animals resulting in poor utilisation of food because of various disabilities. These conditions are important in young pigs which are destined to play their part in breeding units, since significant trouble in this group will ultimately affect the profitability of any breeding enterprise.

Constitutional or non-infectious diseases of the skeletal system include Osteochondrosis (Degenerative Joint Disease), Osteomalacia (Osteoporosis) and Rickets.

Osteochondrosis

This condition is extremely common occurring worldwide and affects young growing pigs causing lameness and joint deformities.

➤ CLINICAL SIGNS

The heaviest pigs in the litter are more likely to be affected than others. Lameness and tentative movements are first seen. The joints soon become stiff and in severe cases the animal is unable to stand. In the older animal if the disease has progressed the condition can interfere with the ability to copulate. Pigs are occasionally noted in the kneeling position due to an inability to stand properly. Arching of the back can also occur.

> **TREATMENT**

1. CALC PHOSPH. This is the main remedy to consider for young pigs. It will stabilise the mineral balance and produce strong bones and muscles in the developing animal. Suggested potency 30c one dose three times per week for four weeks.

2. HECLA LAVA. This remedy has a reputation for producing hardening of bone and preventing subsequent deterioration of the condition. Suggested potency 200c one dose three times per week for four weeks.

3. SILICEA. This remedy acts not unlike the previous one but will probably produce better results in lean or (supposedly) poorly nourished animals. The Tamworth breed may benefit more from this remedy than others. Suggested potency 200c one dose three times per week for six weeks.

*O*steomalacia (Osteoporosis)

This condition affects mainly older animals and assumes economic importance in breeding herds when, if sows become affected, lameness leading to paraplegia or paralysis develops.

> **CLINICAL SIGNS**

Affected animals show rigidity of limbs and eventually are unable to stand. Fractures of bones can occur preceded by crepitus: once the disease has established itself treatment may be ineffective and owners should be encouraged to concentrate on herd prevention. This is based on the remedies

CALC PHOSPH, HECLA LAVA and SILICEA as in OSTEOCHONDROSIS.

Degenerative Joint Disease Associated with Infections

Streptococci, Staphylococci and E. coli can all be implicated in the occurrence of these conditions affecting mainly young piglets. Infection can take place through the umbilicus or via suckling from a carrier sow. Joints become hot and shiny and swelling is pronounced. The umbilicus may also become puffy and oedematous.

▶ **TREATMENT**

Remedies such as RHUS TOX 6c or 1m: ACID SAL 200c: APIS MEL 30c: HEPAR SULPH 30c: BRYONIA 30c and ACTAEA 30c may all be useful in their own way (see chapter on Materia Medica). The concurrent use of the appropriate nosodes should also help, using them in 30c potency once per day for ten days.

Rickets

This deficiency disease is seen from time to time and arises because of an imbalance of the calcium/phosphorus ratio in association with a deficiency of Vitamin D. Once established, the condition is probably beyond treatment and owners are advised to concentrate on prophylactic measures. The remedy CALC PHOSPH 30c should be given as a routine measure to young piglets from one week old to two months, at the rate of one dose twice weekly. Vitamin D can also be used as an accompaniment. This vitamin should be given in organic form and not as a synthetically prepared product.

Weakness of Hooves

Poor growth, brittleness and crackling of hooves in adult animals should be treated with the remedy *SILICEA* in 200c potency giving one dose three times per week for six weeks. This invariably results in the development of healthy horn of hard texture thereby limiting the tendency to further trouble arising.

Foot Rot

This condition can affect pigs up to six months of age if reared on concrete as opposed to wooden flooring. Cracks develop on the wall of the hoof sometimes incorporating the coronary band. Secondary infection leads to the development of ulcerated surfaces which in severe cases can involve the laminal, ultimately affecting deeper structures such as bones and tendons. Neglected cases can lead to septicaemia. Occasionally the sole of the foot as opposed to the wall of the hoof is implicated. The foot rot organism *Fusiformis necrophorus* is often found to be the cause as in sheep and cattle. Laminitis occasionally arises as a sequel to this condition.

➤ **TREATMENT**

1. **SILICEA.** This remedy given as soon as cracks appear on the wall of the hoof will do much to halt the progress of the condition. It will also help heal fistulous tracts. Suggested potency 200c three times per week for four weeks.

2. **KREOSOTUM.** This is a well-proven remedy in the treatment of foot rot when foul-smelling ulcers develop giving rise to the production of crumbly cheese-like horn. Suggested potency 200c twice per week for five weeks.

3. HEPAR SULPH. This remedy may help reduce pain and limit early infection around the coronary band. Suggested potency 1m one dose three times per week for two weeks.

4. PYROGEN. If septicaemic complications develop this remedy should be used in 1m potency one dose three times daily for three days.

5. FUSIFORMIS NOSODE. In 30c potency once per day for ten days this remedy can be used in conjunction with any other remedy.

CHAPTER FOUR

INFERTILITY
and Reproductive Failure

IRREGULARITIES OF THE oestrus cycle are not so common in sows as they are in other species but if there is a history of such the remedy *SEPIA* should be considered as a primary remedy. This remedy regulates the function of the entire genital tract and if necessary can be given in 200c potency one dose per week for three weeks. Sows which show a persistent vaginal discharge which may lead to an inability to conceive should benefit from the remedy *CALC PHOSPH* 30c one dose per day for 21 days. If lack of ovulation is thought to be a factor in conception failure *PULSATILLA* in 200c potency may help giving one dose per week for three weeks. Other ovarian remedies which should be kept in mind and which may be needed are *IODUM, PLATINA* and *PALLADIUM* each in 200c potency and they can be given as for Pulsatilla (see Materia Medica).

Once pregnancy has been established there are two main remedies which should help maintain this viz. *VIBURNUM OPULIS* and *CAULOPHYLLUM*. The former is given early in pregnancy around one month. One dose of 30c three times per week for four weeks. The latter is used in the last month, one dose of 30c three times per week. This remedy should also help ensure a trouble free parturition.

Infertility in the boar is not usually a serious problem but the following remedies may help depending on the actual condition, e.g. poor semen count may respond to the remedy *PITUITARY WHOLE* 30c giving one dose per day for 30 days and repeating this after an interval of two weeks. The remedy *LYCOPODIUM* in 200c potency has proved helpful in animals which show a temporary impotence or loss of libido giving the remedy once daily for 25 days.

Post Partum Complications

1. HAEMORRHAGE. There are a group of remedies which have a bearing on bleeding after parturition, the most important of these being the following: a) *IPECACUANHA* 30c. With this remedy the blood is bright red and comes away in what has been described as a flood. It should be given every hour for four or five doses b) *CROTALUS LORRIDUS* 10m. When blood is lost in a steady drip as opposed to the former remedy it could prove beneficial. Dosage is as for the previous remedy. c) *SABINA* 6c. This remedy appears to be more useful when used after abortions or early farrowing, one dose every two hours for five doses may be needed. d) *ARNICA* 30c. If parturition has proved difficult or prolonged bleeding will be controlled by this remedy giving one dose three times daily for three days. e) *SECALE* 200c. Indications for this is dark (almost black) blood: the remedy is associated with premature farrowing. Dose one three times daily for three days. f) *HAMAMELIS* 30c. Venous bleeding as opposed to arterial calls for this remedy, one dose three times daily for three days. Other remedies which influence post–partum haemorrhage are *MELILOTUS, MILLEFOLIUM, FICUS RELIGIOSA, PHOSPHORUS, USTILLAGO, TEREBINTHINAE* and *TRILLIUM* (see Materia Medica) all in 30c potency.

2. UTERINE PROLAPSE. This not uncommon condition must be dealt with surgically but the remedies *ARNICA*, *SEPIA* and *STAPHISAGRIA* are indicated to help the sow retain the uterus and prevent relapse. As the condition can be looked on as an injury the remedy *ARNICA* in 200c potency should be given, one dose daily for three days, followed by *SEPIA* in the same potency one dose three times per week for two weeks. The remedy *STAPHISAGRIA* is used as a routine after operations and materially aids recovery: it could therefore be indicated in this particular instance, potency 30c one daily for five days.

3. AGALACTIA. This is a fairly common post-partum condition and has been looked at in an earlier chapter (see *E. coli* infection). Non-specific cases of agalactia call for the remedy *URTICA URENS* in high (200c) potency, one daily for six or seven days. *MEDUSA* is another less well known remedy which can be used in this connection using a 30c potency three times daily for five days. To enhance the value of these remedies *PITUITARY WHOLE* 30c is indicated one dose daily for seven days.

4. METRITIS. This potentially serious complication calls for prompt action. Early signs are fever, inappetance, loss of milk, discolouration of skin: uterine discharge may or may not be present. The remedy *ACONITUM* in 10m potency should be given as early as possible one dose every hour for four doses. *PYROGEN* is one of the principal remedies to combat this condition. The main indication for its use is a discrepancy between pulse and temperature. Dosage is one dose of 10m every hour for four doses. It could be repeated daily for three days. *CAULOPHYLLUM* 30c is indicated if there is blood-stained discharge as well.

CHAPTER FIVE

MASTITIS, *and other Affections of the Mammary Glands, including Lactation*

THESE TERMS COVER various disturbances of the mammary glands from simple inflammations and indurations to agalactia. Inflammation of the glands can take the form of a hot tense swelling to a less acute firm induration. Oedema of the glands is frequently present. These complexes are not uncommon in the first day or two after parturition. In nearly all cases presented, mastitis is accompanied by a deficiency or absence of lactation.

➤ ETIOLOGY

There are various causes of this condition depending on whether it is specific or non-specific. In the former the *E. coli* organisms have been incriminated while non-specific causes include oedema of the glands, ketosis and calcium and other mineral deficiencies. Gilts farrowing for the first time occasionally exhibit abnormal behaviour towards the piglets and this appears to have an influence on the glands suppressing the milk flow. Other less commonly encountered causes include infections of the uro-genital tract and various viruses and mycoplasms. It is necessary also to keep in mind the role that nutritional factors could play in the development of the mastitis/agalactia syndrome. Mineral and vitamin deficiencies have also been shown to play an important part.

► TREATMENT

The following remedies all have a part to play depending on the nature of the condition presented and the particular infectious agent involved.

1. BELLADONNA. This remedy is indicated when the glands are hot and tense with the overlying skin warm and shiny. Temperature is usually raised and the sow may exhibit signs of central nervous involvement such as hyper-excitability. Suggested potency 1m one dose every hour for four doses.

2. BRYONIA. Hardness of the drills is a keynote of this remedy. The animal is disinclined to move and if made to do so will quickly revert to a recumbent posture. Suggested potency 30c one dose three times daily for five days.

3. URTICA URENS. This remedy is one of the most important in considering the treatment of lactation problems. When agalactia is the problem the remedy should be used in high potency, e.g. 200c, giving it daily for seven days.

4. PHYTOLACCA. This remedy has a selective action on glandular tissue and can be considered in the treatment of sub-acute or chronic conditions of the mammary glands. Suggested potency 30c daily for fourteen days.

5. E. COLI 30C. This organism is a prime cause of agalactia and although there is a multiplicity of strains of *E. coli* the one that is marketed as *E. coli* (Ainsworths Pharmacy who first developed it) is the one of choice. A potency of 30c should be given daily for seven days and it can be combined with other selected remedies.

6. VITAMIN E. This vitamin is of prime importance in increasing the blood-supply – and thereby oxygen – to the tissues and this acts as a most valuable remedial agent. It can either be used as straight Vit E – marketed as different international units or as low potency, e.g. 1x homoeopathic preparations. Natural Vit E could be given in 250 units daily for two weeks or as 1x potency three times daily for twenty one days.

7. SELENIUM. Deficiency of this mineral should be countered by the use of *SELENIUM* 6c giving it three times daily for twenty one days.

8. MYCOPLASMA NOSODE. If the appropriate organism can be identified it should be given daily in 30c for seven days combined with selected remedies.

To avoid time and repetition of different remedies Belladonna, Bryonia and Urtica Urens are marketed under the name of B.BU.30c.

CHAPTER SIX

PORCINE *Stress Syndrome*

SYMPTOMS OF STRESS in pigs are sometimes manifested in various ways, e.g. tremors of the tail and muscles. Laboured breathing and pale and reddened areas also occur, also cyanosis. Temperature rise accompanies these signs.

➤ **TREATMENT**

Any form of stress should be treated with *ACONITUM.*

Acute symptoms indicate a high potency, e.g. 10m giving one dose every hour for four doses. Less acute symptoms call for a lower potency, e.g. 200c one dose daily for five days or so.

CHAPTER SEVEN

VIRAL *Diseases*

A denoviruses

These viruses have been associated with encephalitis, diarrhoea, kidney infections and pneumonia. Abortions have also been noted.

➤ **TREATMENT**

Pigs succumbing to viral infections causing encephalitis may respond to *BELLADONNA, CICUTA VIROSA, PLUMBUM, CUPRUM MET* or *STRAMONIUM* depending on overall symptoms presented. Remedies which could favourably influence diarrhoea include *ARSENICUM ALBUM, CHINA OFFICINALIS, VERATRUM ALBUM, PODOPHYLLUM* and the bowel nosodes *E. COLI* and *GAERTNER*. Kidney infections are usually associated with secondary invasion of pyogenic bacteria following primary viral invasion. The remedies *HEPAR SULPH* and *E. COLI* may help in these cases. Pneumonia and its complications such as pleurisy are covered by a variety of remedies chief among which are *PHOSPHORUS, ANTIMONIUM TARTARICUM, ANTIMONIUM ARSENICOSUM* and *BRYONIA* among others. Nosodes prepared against specific viruses should provide protection against abortions in combination with remedies such as *VIBURNUM OPULIS* and *CAULOPHYLLUM*.

Potencies of these various remedies should commence at 30c and progress to 1m and 10m if necessary under veterinary supervision.

African Swine Fever

This disease is caused by a DNA virus which affects cells of the reticulo-endothelial system and can be transmitted by ticks of the *Ornithodorus* Spp. It can present as acute, sub-acute (or sub-clinical) and chronic forms.

➤ CLINICAL SIGNS

The acute form is ushered in by a rise in temperature followed by loss of appetite. Anaemic signs may be present while small haemorrhages appear on the skin especially that of the ears and flanks. Sub-clinical and chronic forms which are those normally found in European outbreaks – are associated with pneumonias and abortions. An incubation period covering a period of four to eight days may extend in exceptional cases and outbreaks to nineteen days. This variation is dependent on the virulence of the invading virus. Spread can take place by ticks and by secretions and discharges from mouth and nose leading to viral incorporation of tonsils and other lymphoid tissues from where spread to the blood, spleen and bone-marrow takes place.

Even if treatment were permitted in those countries where this disease is endemic this would in all probability be ineffective and uneconomic. Protection by nosode using the potentised virus in 30c potency is a possible means of protection.

This disease is notifiable in the United Kingdom under the Diseases of Animals Acts and Orders.

Blue Eye Disease

This disease is caused by a paramyxovirus and is characterised by reproductive disorders, corneal opacities and disturbances of the central nervous system. Discolouration of the skin of the ears is sometimes seen.

➤ **CLINICAL SIGNS**

The owner or attendant is first alerted by disturbances of the central nervous system in farrowing sows followed by still-births and the appearance of corneal opacity in weaned pigs. Very young piglets are especially susceptible. An early rise in temperature is followed by prostration. The coat becomes rough and general nervous signs appear which tend to become progressively severe, muscular rigidity and hind-leg weakness being typical signs. Hyperexcitability occurs in a proportion of piglets.

Involvement of eye structures such as conjunctivitis and lachrymation is evident in many outbreaks, followed by corneal discolouration and opacity. Older pigs exhibit less involvement of the central nervous system, but respiratory signs such as coughing are more prominent. Corneal opacity is also a feature of infection in the older pig. Sows and gilts in the majority of cases become infertile, manifested by failure to conceive while in-pig sows suffer abortions and still-births. Boars can also become infected showing testicular swelling (usually one sided).

➤ **TREATMENT**

1. **BELLADONNA.** This remedy may be useful in controlling central nervous system involvement and limiting muscle rigidity. Suggested potency 200c one dose daily for ten days.

2. AGARICUS. In-coordination and ataxia affecting the hind-limbs should benefit from this remedy. Suggested potency 30c daily for fourteen days.

3. SILICEA. This remedy is indicated in cases of corneal opacity. Suggested potency 200c one dose three times per week for three weeks.

4. CURARE. Muscular rigidity in general is associated with this remedy. Suggested potency 30c one dose per day for fourteen days.

5. CAULOPHYLLUM. Still births and late abortions are associated with this remedy which has a proven value in these connections. Suggested potency 30c one dose twice weekly for the last two months of pregnancy.

6. BRYONIA. Respiratory involvement in the older pig may benefit from this remedy. Suggested potency 30c one dose twice daily for fourteen days. One of the keynotes of this remedy is worse for any movement, the patient preferring to remain still.

7. PHOSPHORUS. Rapid breathing dependent on consolidation of lung tissue in pneumonia indicates this remedy. Suggested potency 1m–10m one dose three times daily for three days depending on the severity of the particular infection.

Border Disease

The incriminating viral agent associated with this disease is closely related to the virus which causes Mucosal Disease in cattle. All ages of pigs are susceptible to infection but particularly sows in which infertility problems occur such as small litters, still births and abortions. Systemic signs include conjunctivitis, skin discolouration such as bluish discolouration of the tips of the ears, skin haemhorrages, diarrhoea and arthritis. Clinical signs are particularly prominent if sows become infected during the first third of pregnancy.

➤ **TREATMENT**

1. **ARGENTUM NITRICUM.** This is a remedy which has given good results in cases of conjunctivitis. Suggested potency 30c one dose daily for fourteen days.

2. **VERATRUM ALB.** This is one of the remedies which may help control diarrhoea. Stools are often described as "rice water". Suggested potency 30c one dose daily for fourteen days.

3. **CHINA OFF.** Dehydration as a result of excessive diarrhoea and loss of body fluid will benefit from this remedy. Suggested potency 6c one dose three times daily for seven days.

4. **RHUS TOX 1M.** Those cases which develop arthritis should be helped by this remedy. Suggested potency 1m one dose daily for ten days.

5. **VIBURNUM OPULIS.** This is a remedy which is used to help prevent abortions in the first third of pregnancy. Suggested potency 30c one dose three times per week for three weeks.

6. **CAULOPHYLLUM.** Later abortions will be influenced by this remedy and it should also help sows to carry their litters to full term and eliminate still births. Suggested potency 30c one dose twice per week for the last six weeks of pregnancy.

> **PREVENTION**

A nosode prepared from the virus can be used as a prophylactic measure using a 30c potency.

*C*ongenital Tremors Disease

This widespread viral disease affects piglets at birth or shortly after, especially those from gilts rather than from older animals. Subsequent litters from affected gilts and sows are rarely affected.

> **CLINICAL SIGNS**

Tremors are evident on both sides of the body.

Muscle contractions vary in intensity from mild tremors over the flank or hind legs to more violent seizures leading to difficulty in walking. These tremors and spasms tend to disappear after a few weeks. Muscular spasms can be induced by external stimuli such as loud noises or excitement. Occasionally pigs are found in a sitting position with legs spread out under the body.

> **TREATMENT**

1. **CUPRUM METALLICUM.** This remedy has a proven record in the treatment of muscular cramps and seizures. Suggested potency 30c one dose three times daily for seven days.

2. **CURARE.** Rigidity and stiffening of muscles leading to a semi-paralytic state should benefit from this remedy, especially when the lower back is affected. Suggested potency 30c one dose daily for fourteen days.

3. **STRYCHNINUM.** Muscular twitchings and hyper-stimulation of nerve endings are associated with this remedy. Suggested potency 1m one dose daily for ten days.

4. CONIUM. This is a useful remedy to control these cases which are presented with weakness of the hind limbs. Suggested potency 30c one dose daily for fourteen days. Ascending potencies up to 10m may be needed to follow depending on response.

5. LATHYRUS. If the previous remedy fails to give satisfactory results as is possible in some cases this remedy may prove useful. Suggested potency 1m one dose daily for ten days.

> **PREVENTION**

A nosode based on the causative virus or infective material should be used as a prophylactic measure in 30c potency.

Cytomegalovirus Infection

This viral disease is seen in many different countries and occurs in different age groups. Very young pigs can be infected through the placenta and as well as neo-nates being affected, still births and mummified foetuses are not uncommon sequelae.

> **CLINICAL SIGNS**

Rhinitis with or without pneumonic complications is not uncommon. Infected pigs of older age groups may show no clinical signs but new-born piglets suffer from high temperature and die fairly quickly. In-pig sows become listless and depressed. Some affected piglets are anaemic developing swelling of hind-leg joints.

> **TREATMENT**

1. HYDRASTIS. This is a remedy which is associated with catarrhal inflammation and should be of benefit in the treatment of early cases of rhinitis. Suggested potency 30c one dose daily for fourteen days.

2. PHOSPHORUS. If pneumonia supervenes this remedy which has given good results in many cases may prove useful. Suggested potency 1m one dose three times per week for four weeks.

3. APIS MELLIFICA. Joint swellings are associated with this remedy and it should be considered in early cases of synovitis or bursitis. Suggested potency 30c one dose three times daily for seven days.

4. CAULOPHYLLUM. This remedy will be of benefit in controlling the tendency to abortions and still births. Suggested potency 30c one dose twice weekly for the last four weeks of pregnancy.

Encephalomyocarditis Virus Infection

An agent of the *Picornovirus* family is associated with this condition. It leads to reproductive disorders in sows and high mortality in new-born piglets.

➤ **CLINICAL SIGNS**

The condition is invariably acute causing death by heart failure. Nervous signs also are seen such as trembling, uncoordination and paralysis. Respiratory complications are evidenced by difficulty in breathing. A high temperature is a feature of the disease in young pigs while older animals may show few acute symptoms. Abortions occur in pregnant sows with also still births and reduced numbers of litters.

➤ **PREVENTION**

As treatment is likely to be ineffective in most cases, prophylactic measures should be considered. A nosode could be made from any infective material and used in 30c potency.

*E*nterovirus

The viruses implicated in enteric diseases of pigs may cause different clinical symptoms which include disturbance of reproductive function, pneumonia and various bowel conditions. Affections of the central nervous system are also commonly encountered manifesting themselves as diseases such as Teschen Disease – a polioencephalomyelitis and Talfan Disease causing extensive paresis.

➤ ETIOLOGY
These conditions are associated with invasion of *Picornovirus*.

➤ CLINICAL SIGNS
A. Polioencephalomyelitis. This condition is sometimes referred to as Teschen Disease manifested to begin with by a rise in temperature and loss of appetite. Peripheral nervous complications may follow, e.g. unsteady gait which may proceed to convulsions followed by coma. These conditions are exacerbated by exposure to light or external stimuli.

In the enzootic (paresis) form – Talfan Disease – mainly young piglets are affected but progression to paralysis is uncommon.

B. Reproductive involvement. This may lead to mummified foetuses and still births and infertility in general. Premonitory or prodromal signs may be absent.

C. Pneumonia accompanied by heart disease. In these cases symptoms may be mild or difficult to ascertain.

Teschen disease is notifiable in the United Kingdom under the Diseases of Animals Acts and Orders.

Encephalomyelitis Virus

This particular virus, thought to be a coronavirus, is associated with encephalomyelitis leading to retarded growth. The virus is believed to spread by natural infection.

➤ CLINICAL SIGNS

There are two main manifestations of this condition depending on which body systems are involved viz. 1) an encephalomyelitis affecting piglets under four weeks of age and 2) a more chronic form involving the alimentary tract where vomiting and diarrhoea develop after an incubation period of up to one week. Young pigs (under four weeks) are at risk exhibiting vomiting and diarrhoea. Grinding of the teeth is a common accompaniment. Arching of the back in affected pigs is frequently seen. Rapid loss of condition follows due to the loss of food consequent on persistent vomiting. Difficult breathing accompanied by cyanosis of the skin precede death. Older pigs exhibit the same symptoms but eventually die after severe wasting. Sows may develop immunity and pass this on to their offspring.

➤ TREATMENT

This is likely to be ineffective but the remedies *PHOSPHORUS* and *ARSEN ALB.* could be used to control excessive vomiting and diarrhoea in less acute cases.

➤ PREVENTION

A nosode prepared against the particular virus might provide a degree of protection in herds which are at risk.

Swine Fever (Hog Cholera)

This is a viral disease which is highly contagious. Acute, sub-acute and chronic forms are recognised. Many cases can appear as atypical. Virulent infections are associated with high morbidity and deaths. If the virus is of lower virulence signs may be mild and in some cases may go unnoticed.

➤ ETIOLOGY

The particular virus belongs to the same family which includes the virus of Bovine Viral Diarrhoea – viz. *Pestivirus*.

➤ CLINICAL SIGNS

Early signs of infection in a herd show affected pigs to be drowsy and listless. Arching of the back is seen. Loss of appetite is a normal feature. A rise in temperature occurs in all cases. Early in infection conjunctivitis occurs producing a sticky discharge which may be severe enough to cause the eyelids to stick together. Early constipation in the pyrexic stage is followed by diarrhoea of a greyish or yellowish colour. Affected pigs are seen huddled together presumably in an attempt to keep warm. Vomiting and convulsions follow in some cases; as the disease progresses pigs become ataxic and eventually become recumbent due to paralysis. Purplish discolouration of the skin of various areas precedes death.

This disease in the U.K. is notifiable under the Diseases of Animals Acts and Orders and treatment is forbidden accordingly. The disease is mentioned here in an attempt to provide the owner or attendant with a rough guide to the cardinal symptoms.

Porcine Epidemic Diarrhoea

Feeder pigs in recent years have been reported suffering from gastro-enteritis similar to the specific disease Transmissible Gastro Enteritis but investigation established the cause to be associated with a different virus. In the case of epidemic diarrhoea young suckling pigs (under one month of age) are not affected.

➤ **ETIOLOGY**

A coronavirus is thought to be implicated.

➤ **CLINICAL SIGNS**

A watery diarrhoea affects pigs of all ages particularly older groups resulting in deaths after a period of three to four days. Depression and lack of appetite are early signs. Abdominal pain manifested by colicky signs is a common feature.

➤ **TREATMENT**

1. ACONITUM. If the early symptoms are noticed in time this remedy may help to limit the progression of the disease. Suggested potency 10m one dose every hour for four doses.

2. VERATRUM ALB. This is just one of the remedies which could help in cases of diarrhoea. Stools are described as watery and greenish. Suggested potency 30c twice daily for five days.

3. CHINA OFF. The weakness associated with loss of fluid after diarrhoea will benefit from this remedy. Suggested potency 6c one dose three times daily for five days.

4. NUX VOMICA. Loss of appetite may be helped by this remedy using a potency of 1m three times daily for seven days.

5. COLOCYNTHIS. Abdominal colic is associated with this remedy. Suggested potency 1m one dose every hour for four doses.

➤ **PREVENTION**

A nosode could be prepared from any affected tissue or discharge and used in a 30c potency. This could also be used in treatment along with selected remedies.

Porcine Parvovirus

This virus affects in-pig sows when they are exposed to infection in the first three months of pregnancy. Foetuses may become infected because of transference of infection via the placenta. Pigs other than in-pig gilts or sows appear to be unaffected.

➤ ETIOLOGY

A virus of the *Parvovirus* family is implicated.

➤ CLINICAL SIGNS

The main indication that anything is amiss is reproductive failure among sows. Mummified foetuses are a common feature of the disease. There may also be abortions while foetuses which are carried to full term are born dead.

➤ TREATMENT

1. VIBURNUM OPULIS. This remedy is associated with miscarriages in the early stages of pregnancy. Suggested potency 30c one dose three times per week for two weeks after the first month.

2. CAULOPHYLLUM. Later stages of pregnancy are covered by this remedy. It should be used to prevent miscarriages or abortions in the last four weeks of pregnancy. Suggested potency 30c twice weekly for the last four weeks.

➤ PREVENTION

The remedy *SEPIA* in 200c potency could be helpful in regulating the genital tract and together with the appropriate nosode could be instrumental in limiting infection in herds.

*A*ujesky's Disease – Pseudorabies

This viral disease is associated with a member of the Herpes Virus family, and pigs are the only natural hosts of this virus.

➤ CLINICAL SIGNS

Young pigs are commonly affected when respiratory and nervous symptoms predominate. Respiratory complications are more often seen in older pigs while younger animals are more likely to be affected by the nervous form. Abortions in sows are early signs. Feeding pigs become anorexic; this loss of appetite being accompanied by listlessness and an appearance of depression. Coughing develops when respiratory involvement supervenes. Loss of balance and convulsions may also occur. The incubation period is two to four days. Neonatal and suckling pigs exhibit nervous signs such as ataxia, vomiting and diarrhoea. Weaned pigs (three to nine weeks); in this age group symptoms are less severe and include early rise of temperature and loss of appetite. Involvement of the respiratory system is manifested by sneezing and coughing. Loss of weight is normally encountered. Secondary infections are common leading to complications of varying kinds. Pigs remain stunted while lateral deviation of the head is often seen in older or fattening pigs. Respiratory involvement is the main sign. Central nervous symptoms are less common but are frequently seen, and consist of trembling and convulsions. Occasionally recovery takes place after the temperature returns to normal. In adult pigs respiratory symptoms predominate while in-pig sows may abort or carry their foetuses to full term when they are born dead. Earlier pregnancies sometimes end as resorption of foetuses takes place.

This disease is notifiable in the United Kingdom under the Diseases of Animals Acts and Orders.

Porcine Rotavirus

Viruses of this group are associated with gastro-enteritis and diarrhoea and are also capable of causing enzootic diarrhoea.

> ## CLINICAL SIGNS

In general young piglets which are deprived of colostrum are susceptible. After an incubation period of twelve to twenty four hours loss of appetite sets in accompanied by intermittent vomiting: profuse yellowish-white diarrhoea follows, leading to dehydration. Older pigs are less likely to be affected by dehydration and diarrhoea. The majority of adult animals are immune to these viruses, but natural infection is very common in the younger age groups.

> ## TREATMENT

1. ARSENICUM ALBUM. This remedy should be considered to control early vomiting and may also help stop any progression to enteritis and diarrhoea. Suggested potency 1m one dose every hour for four doses.

2. VERATRUM ALB. This is an excellent remedy to help control diarrhoea, the stools assuming a "rice water" appearance. Suggested potency 30c one dose three times daily for seven days.

3. CAMPHORA. Dehydration due to excessive loss of fluid should be helped by this remedy. Symptoms may come on suddenly and progress rapidly. Suggested potency 30c one dose every hour for four doses, followed by three times daily for a further three days.

4. CHINA OFF. This remedy is also useful to control dehydration but symptoms are less severe than in the previous remedy. Suggested potency 6c one dose three times daily for seven days.

5. Phosphorus. If vomiting is the more prominent symptom as opposed to diarrhoea this remedy may prove useful. Suggested potency 200c one dose three times daily for five days.

6. Rotavirus Nosode. This could be combined with any selected remedy using a potency of 30c daily for five days.

➤ **Prevention**

The same nosode should be used on a herd basis to provide protection.

Porcine Reovirus

This group of viruses has been shown to inhabit the respiratory and reproductive tracts of healthy pigs but it is unclear whether they act as pathogenic agents or are merely commensals. Reoviruses are widely distributed among pig units leading to a variety of clinical signs including mild fever, sneezing and loss of appetite. Listlessness is followed by diarrhoea. Sows are liable to produce still born and weak piglets, while other foetuses may be born in a viable state.

➤ **Treatment**

Early rise in temperature should indicate *ACONITUM* and this remedy in high (10m) potency may help prevent disease taking a more severe form. One dose every hour for four doses should suffice.

1. Pulsatilla. This remedy may help control early respiratory signs such as sneezing. Suggested potency 30c one dose three times daily for two days.

2. NUX VOMICA. Loss of appetite may be helped by this remedy in 1m potency, one dose three times per day for three days.

3. ARSENICUM ALB. This remedy has proved successful in controlling diarrhoea. Stools tend to become evil smelling and dark, while the affected animal is thirsty for small quantities of water at frequent intervals.

4. CAULOPHYLLUM. This is a well-proven remedy to control complications in later pregnancy and has given good results in trials where the incidence of still births was greatly reduced after its use. Suggested potency 30c.

Swine Influenza. Hog 'Flu

This is an acute infectious disease affecting the respiratory system and is caused by a specific virus called *Influenza A*. The disease is sudden in onset and affects the respiratory tract mainly. Recovery is the rule except where pneumonia supervenes. Movement of animals may lead to rapid spread and many farms can be affected simultaneously. Most animals in a herd in any given outbreak are likely to be affected. Variations in external temperatures, e.g. cold nights following warm days may trigger an outbreak as also will exposure to damp.

► CLINICAL SIGNS

This is a herd disease and all animals are likely to show the same response to infection. Onset is sudden followed by an incubation period of one to three days. Loss of appetite is an early sign while prostration leads to affected pigs huddling together. There is disinclination to move. Breathing becomes laboured and open-mouthed. Progression to pneumonia is indicated by the severity of the respiratory symptoms including abdominal breathing. If animals are made to move this brings on coughing which is harsh and dry. Temperature remains high while outward signs include conjunctivitis and nasal discharge. Although most members of the herd will probably be affected, mortality is low except possibly in very young piglets. Reproductive and neonatal problems may arise such as abortions and weak litters. Inability of sows and gilts to conceive could be a complicating factor.

➤ TREATMENT

1. ACONITUM. This remedy should be given as soon as early symptoms appear. A potency of 10m is indicated one dose every hour for four doses.

2. GELSEMIUM. Listlessness and prostration indicate the need for this remedy. Suggested potency 200c one dose every hour for three doses, followed by one three times daily for two days.

3. BRYONIA. Disinclination to move is the keynote for the use of this remedy. Any movement brings on coughing and distress. Suggested potency 30c one dose three times daily for five days.

4. PHOSPHORUS. Severe cases with pneumonia complications leading to mouth breathing and harsh dry cough should be helped by this remedy. Suggested potency 200c one dose twice daily for two days, followed by 1m one dose daily for four days.

5. DULCAMARA. If the condition arises as a result of exposure to cold nights after warm days this remedy will prove very useful: also after exposure to damp. Suggested potency 200c one dose twice daily for five days.

6. CAULOPHYLLUM. As in other conditions which lead to reproductive problems this remedy will be indicated. Suggested potency 30c one dose twice per week for the last four weeks of pregnancy.

7. SEPIA. If sows and gilts exhibit an inability to conceive after recovering from infection this remedy in 200c potency will prove useful, giving one dose per week for three weeks.

➤ **PREVENTION**
Swine Influenza nosode should be considered to prevent disease, and could also be combined with other remedies in treatment.

*S*wine Pox

This disease is caused by a specific virus given the name of Swine Pox virus to distinguish it from other pox viruses, e.g. vaccinia which is relatively uncommon in pigs. The disease is found in most countries and is invariably associated with poor sanitation and also with intensive breeding programmes. Deaths from swine pox are uncommon but the condition can affect the majority of pigs in any one outbreak.

➤ **CLINICAL SIGNS**
The usual signs of early infection are the same as in pox diseases in other species viz. beginning with the papular stage and progressing to vesicle, pustule and finally scab formation. The vesicular stage is frequently ill-defined. The course of the disease runs roughly from three to four weeks. Swelling of lymph glands has been reported in some out-breaks. Young animals are more severely affected than mature pigs and may exhibit lesions over the entire body surface. Older pigs (around four months or so) show lesions mainly on the hairless parts of the body. In adult stock

lesions may appear on the udder and vulva of sows and gilts along with involvement of ears and snout of both sexes.

➤ **TREATMENT**

1. **ANTIMONIUM CRUDUM.** This is a very useful remedy which has given good results in the early stages of this infection. Given as soon as the papular stage is seen it will limit the progression to further stages. Suggested potency 6c one dose three times daily for three days.

2. **ACIDUM NITRICUM.** Lesions around the snout should respond to treatment by this remedy. Suggested potency 200c one dose three times per week for two weeks. It should also be helpful in sows and gilts with vulval lesions.

3. **CALC FLUOR.** Pigs which show swelling of lymph glands may benefit from this remedy. Suggested potency 30c one dose daily for ten days.

4. **VARIOLINUM.** This nosode – although not specifically derived from Swine Pox virus – will prove useful combined with any of the other selected remedies. Suggested potency 30c one dose daily for seven days.

➤ **PREVENTION**

The same nosode (or Swine Pox nosode if available) should be considered on a herd basis. Specific Swine Pox nosode could be made from vesicular or pustular material.

Swine Vesicular Disease

This condition is caused by a virus belonging to the family Picornoviridae. It is capable of affecting man as well as pigs. It is only moderately infectious. Spread of the disease is caused by contact with infected pigs and by excretions: also by contaminated meat products. The disease is important because of its clinical similarity to Foot and Mouth Disease.

➤ CLINICAL SIGNS

A preliminary rise in temperature is followed by the appearance of vesicles around the coronary band. The pyrexia may last up to five days. Vesicles appear on the snout from where extension to lips, tongue and pharynx takes place. Lesions are also seen in the interdigital clefts and soft tissues of the foot. Salivation is an invariable sign, but the specific 'smacking' sound associated with lesions in Foot and Mouth Disease are generally absent. Nursing sows may show lesions on the teats. Rupture of vesicles yields a serous fluid followed by detachment of epithelium leaving a reddened area. Separation of hoof structures has been reported. Rapid spread from pig to pig is likely but deaths are uncommon except possibly in very young stock.

This Disease is notifiable in the United Kingdom under the Diseases of Animals Acts and Orders.

Vesicular Exanthema

This condition is confined to pigs and is associated with a virus belonging to the *Calici* family. It is moderately contagious and is spread by contact. Cells which become infected lose their substance and develop necrosis preceded by oedema. Spread within the body may result in inflammation of various lymph glands leading to a generalised spread of virus within the body.

➤ CLINICAL SIGNS

These are roughly the same as in other vesicular diseases and only laboratory examination can determine which particular virus is responsible for any particular outbreak.

➤ **PREVENTION**

A nosode could be given on a herd basis as in other diseases.

Foot and Mouth Disease

The earliest sign of this disease in a pig unit is a rise in temperature which can be severe in virulent outbreaks. The animal presents a picture of depression accompanied by loss of appetite. Epithelial tissue becomes paler than normal before vesicles develop. These then occur on the snout, feet and inside the mouth. After a day or so these vesicles rupture leaving a reddened area which becomes denuded of epithelium. Vesicular lesions also develop around the coronary band and in the interdigital cleft leading in severe cases to separation of the hoof. This disease in pigs invariably takes a severe form.

Swine Vesicular Disease and Vesicular Stomatitis

These two diseases present pictures which are clinically indistinguishable from Foot & Mouth Disease and it is extremely important to determine that they are separate entities in order to eliminate the possibility of Foot & Mouth Disease. This is done by laboratory tests.

These three diseases are notifiable under the Diseases of Animal Acts & Orders and they are mentioned here in order to acquaint pig owners with the salient features of the disease.

Transmissible Gastro-Enteritis

This condition is frequently referred to as T.G.E., and is a highly contagious disease affecting piglets under two weeks of age. Deaths are invariably high in any one outbreak. Older animals, although they may become infected, rarely suffer severe complications. Farrowing time poses the greatest risk of this infection being passed to young piglets. Older pigs may show only loss of appetite and mild diarrhoea. When piglets have survived to one month of age deaths are less common. The virus is associated with the coronavirus group and outbreaks are more often seen in the winter months.

➤ CLINICAL SIGNS

After an incubation period of eighteen hours to three days occasional vomiting occurs followed by a watery yellowish diarrhoea. Affected animals soon lose weight and dehydration develops. Rapid spread of the condition leads to a high mortality in any one outbreak. Diarrhoea is profuse and faeces may contain undigested milk. Mortality is related to the age of the pig, older animals being less likely to die. Diarrhoea which is usually mild, together with loss of appetite, are typical of infection in this older age group. Lactating sows experience loss of milk.

➤ TREATMENT

1. *VERATRUM ALB. 30c, CAMPHORA 30c, ALOE 30c* and *PULSATILLA 30c* are remedies which may help alleviate the diarrhoea and thereby ward off dehydration. This is particularly true of the remedy *CAMPHORA*. (See section on Materia Medica for indications for each remedy.)

2. CHINA OFFICINALIS. This is an essential remedy in treatment and will help restore strength after loss of body fluid. Suggested potency 6c one dose three times per day for five days.

➤ PREVENTION

Because of the severity of this disease occurring around farrowing time the use of T.G.E. nosode should be considered. In 30c potency it should be administered to in-pig sows during the last month of pregnancy one dose three times per week. This should be supplemented by giving the nosode to each piglet at birth, one dose three times daily for five days.

Porcine Reproductive and Respiratory Disease

This condition is also known as *Blue Ear Disease* in Britain. It is caused by an R.N.A. virus and produces complications in the reproductive and respiratory systems. Pigs of any age are at risk but the principal economic effects are seen in the reproductive system of pregnant sows. Any or all of the following manifestations of disease may arise viz. abortions, still births, premature farrowing and weak or mummified piglets. Respiratory disease in growing pigs is more likely to be seen in herds which are not concerned with breeding. Secondary infections may lead to deaths in some outbreaks. Pigs are at risk from other infected animals but droplet infection can also take place. Boars can transmit the infection at coitus.

➤ **CLINICAL SIGNS**

Early signs are not unlike those seen in influenza, viz anorexia and conjunctivitis. Blue or cyanotic skin changes sometimes occur on the extremities viz ears, teats and the lower aspect of limbs. Growing or post-weaning pigs develop pneumonia. Abortions, still births, mummified and weak piglets occur in breeding herds. Infertility in sows and boars may follow infection. Coughing and laboured breathing are normal signs in young animals. Diarrhoea in piglets has been noticed together with oedema of facial structures. Piglets around a week old can become ill about five days after exposure to the virus.

> **TREATMENT**

1. ACONITUM. If given early this remedy may prevent the disease symptoms progressing too far. Suggested potency 10m one dose every hour for four doses.

2. ARGENTUM NITRICUM. Conjunctivitis should respond to this remedy in 30c potency giving one dose three times daily for five days.

3. LACHESIS. This remedy has proved useful in treating cyanotic skin lesions more especially when they appear on the left side of the body. Suggested potency 30c one dose three times daily for five days.

4. BRYONIA. Coughing in young animals indicates this remedy; affected pigs are reluctant to move. Suggested potency 30c one dose three times daily for five days.

5. PHOSPHORUS. Established cases of pneumonia may need this remedy. Breathing is heavy and distressed, and of the abdominal type. Suggested potency 10m one dose every hour for four doses followed by one daily for three days.

6. APIS. This remedy may be needed to control facial oedema if it is severe. Suggested potency 6c one dose three times daily for four days.

7. VIBURNUM OPULIS. Early abortions (eight to ten weeks) may be prevented by the use of this remedy. Suggested potency 30c one dose three times per week for three weeks.

8. CAULOPHYLLUM. This is the main remedy to consider to help reduce the incidence of late abortions, still births and weak piglets. Suggested potency 30c one dose twice weekly for the last five weeks of pregnancy.

➤ PREVENTION

A nosode made from viral material including discharge etc. could prove useful in limiting the disease on a herd basis.

CHAPTER EIGHT

BACTERIAL *Diseases*

Pleuropneumonia Associated with Actinobacillus spp.

This disease is caused by a bacterium known as *Actinobacillus pleuropneumonia*, also referred to a *Haemophilus pleuropneumonia*. The disease is widely distributed causing large numbers of deaths in affected herds. Survivors of acute outbreaks become carriers, the bacteria locating in necrotic lung tissue and tonsils. All ages of pigs are susceptible. Spread of the infection is airborne and transmission takes place by contact or by droplet infection. The highest incidence of the disease occurs among feeding pigs.

➤ CLINICAL SIGNS

The incubation period may last from a few days up to three weeks. The disease itself may be per-acute, acute or chronic. Per-acute cases die suddenly or exhibit illness preceded by a rise in temperature, diarrhoea and vomiting. There may be little or no respiratory signs although extreme difficulty in breathing precedes deaths together with frothy blood-stained mucus from mouth and nostrils. Neo-natal piglets develop septicaemia leading to rapid death.

In the acute form a rise in temperature develops among different groups of pigs. Loss of appetite is followed by an appearance of depression together with coughing and difficult breathing. Cyanosis due to involvement of cardiac muscle may take place.

Sub-acute or chronic forms may follow the acute stage. Temperature usually remains normal. Loss of appetite, coughing and arthritis have all been reported in various outbreaks while chronic abscesses develop in different parts of the body.

> ## TREATMENT

1. ACONITUM. This remedy should be given as soon as early signs appear. Suggested potency 10m one dose every hour for four doses.

2. ARSENICUM ALBUM. Diarrhoea and vomiting could be contained by the use of this remedy. Suggested potency 1m one dose twice daily for five days.

3. ECHINACEA. Septicaemic involvement in young pigs may be controlled by this remedy. Suggested potency 3c one dose three times daily for seven days.

4. PHOSPHORUS. This remedy should be beneficial in controlling respiratory symptoms associated with acute cases. Suggested potency 30c twice daily for five days.

5. ACIDUM SALICYLICUM. If arthritis develops as in some chronic states this remedy may prove useful. Suggested potency 200c one dose three times per week for four weeks.

6. SILICEA. If abscesses tend to appear in chronic states this remedy will prove useful. Suggested potency 30c one dose daily for seven days.

> **PREVENTION**

A nosode could be made from infected material and given on a herd basis as in other conditions.

*A*nthrax

This disease is not particularly important in the context of pig medicine as the species is relatively resistant to infection. However outbreaks have been noted from time to time. The disease is important from the viewpoint of transmission to the human population and pigs may act as reservoirs of infection in this connection.

The causative organism is *B. anthracis* which is a sporulating organism which can remain latent in the soil in spore form. Infection through wounds from contaminated soil can lead to the establishment of disease. Soils which have been heavily manured are more likely to lead to infection than those which have not been treated in this way. Bone meal imported from countries where the disease is enzootic is an important source of infection containing as it does in many cases spores of the bacillus.

> **CLINICAL SIGNS**

Deaths among pigs may be the only early sign that something is wrong in the herd. Blood examination will yield proof of infection. Three distinct forms of the disease are recognised viz. pharyngeal, intestinal and septicaemic. Infection may localise in the lymph nodes of the tonsils: or infection may progress to the intestines. Oedema of the neck area is a feature of pharyngeal complication. Rise in temperature is variable while difficult breathing, depression and inappetance occur together with vomiting. Intestinal infection leads to digestive disturbances such as lack of appetite and dysentery. Septicaemia follows after the introduction of the bacteria into the blood stream, resulting in rapid death.

This disease is notifiable under the Diseases of Animals Acts and Orders which forbids treatment. The cardinal symptoms have been described as a guide to owners and stockmen.

A trophic Rhinitis

This is a contagious disease which is widespread in distribution. There are two causative agents 1) *Bordetella bronchiseptica* which is associated with the non-progressive form of the disease and 2) *Pasteurella multicoda* relating to the progressive form. Both types affect the turbinate bones of the nose leading to distortion of the nasal structures. The disease can lead to poor growth among fattening pigs. The severity of the disease is dependent on the virulence of the invading organism and the amount of bacterial toxin absorbed.

➤ CLINICAL SIGNS

These usually occur in pigs in ages from one to three months. In baby pigs snuffling and sneezing are early signs. These symptoms may become continuous as the animal grows. A serous exudate followed by a muco-purulent discharge follows. If bleeding from the nostrils occurs this is invariably one sided. After prolonged sneezing, detached portions of turbinate bone may be seen in nasal discharges. Deformity of nasal and facial structures is a constant feature. The upper jaw becomes shortened in relation to the lower, while the facial skin develops folds. Lateral deviation of the snout is seen in the majority of cases. Occlusion of the lachrymal duct leads to staining of the facial skin due to discharges. There is a general retardation of growth and an inability to utilise feed.

➤ Treatment

1. Aurum metallicum. This remedy has a well documented record in the treatment of degenerative bone disease affecting the nasal structures and is well worth trying in the early stages of this infection. Suggested potency 30c one dose daily for twenty one days.

2. Phosphorus. Haemorrhages accompanying nasal discharges call for this remedy. It will also be of use in necrotic conditions of the nasal bones. Suggested potency 200c one dose three times daily for four weeks.

3. Silicea. Degeneration of turbinate bones followed by shedding of tissue may be helped by this remedy. Suggested potency 200c one dose three times per week for three weeks.

4. Kali bichromicum. If discharges are predominantly purulent this remedy should help. Discharges are yellowish and stringy. Suggested potency 30c one dose daily for seven to ten days.

5. Pulsatilla. Early signs of sneezing and snuffling in young pigs could be favourably influenced by this remedy. Suggested potency 30c one dose daily for seven days.

➤ Prevention

Nosodes prepared against the particular agents responsible for disease should be used on a herd basis employing a 30c potency.

Bordetellosis

This condition is associated with infection by an organism called *Bordetella bronchiseptica* which colonises the nasal passages causing inflammatory changes in the nasal mucosa and also lesions in the turbinate bones. The disease is wide-spread where large pig units exist. Spread from pig to pig is by droplet infection. Sows can be a major source of infection to young suckling pigs.

➤ **CLINICAL SIGNS**

Sneezing and snuffling among groups of young pigs is an early sign. This is particularly so at weaning time. Catarrhal nasal discharge at first clear and later becoming muco-purulent follows soon after. The younger the animal the more severe are the symptoms which develop. Young pigs – around a week old – develop bronchopneumonia manifested by dyspnoea and a whooping type of cough. This form of pneumonia does not affect older pigs. Infection in any particular herd is invariably high and deaths occur in the majority of those affected.

➤ **TREATMENT**

1. ACONITUM. If signs are noticed early enough this reme-dy should be used. Suggested potency 10m one dose every hour for three doses.

2. PULSATILLA. Sneezing and snuffling should be relieved by the use of this remedy. Suggested potency 30c one dose twice daily for seven days.

3. SAMBUCUS. Catarrhal and muco-purulent discharges call for this remedy. Suggested potency 30c one dose daily for ten days.

4. KALI BICHROMICUM. If discharges progress to a more chronic stage producing yellow stringy material this remedy should help. Suggested potency 30c one dose daily for ten days.

5. ANTIMONIUM TARTARICUM. Mild cases of broncho-pneumonia in young pigs associated with a moist cough may be helped by this remedy. Suggested potency 30c one dose three times daily for seven days.

6. DROSERA. More severe forms of lung involvement manifested by a whooping type of cough calls for this remedy. Suggested potency 30c three times daily for seven days.

> **PREVENTION**

A nosode prepared against the causative agent should be used on a herd basis.

Brucellosis

This disease is caused by an organism named *Brucella suis* and occurs in most countries where pig rearing takes place on a large scale. Infection is transmitted to susceptible pigs by contact with infected stock or contaminated discharges, especially those from the alimentary and genital tracts. Suckling pigs can become infected via their dams. Aborted foetuses and foetal membranes are a major source of spread. The disease is classed as venereal in that gilts and sows are at risk from an infected boar.

> **CLINICAL SIGNS**

In the acute stages of the infection bacteraemia occurs which can last several weeks. Classic manifestations are abortion and infertility in sows, testicular swellings in the boar together with posterior paralysis and lameness in both sexes. Abortions can occur at any time during gestation and are highest in sows and gilts which have been infected via the genital tract at breeding time. Vaginal discharge may be absent if abortions take place early in pregnancy. Genital infection tends to persist more in boars leading to swelling of one or both testicles together with swelling of lymph glands, followed by a chronic infertility. Occasionally in a percentage of boars infection does not interfere with breeding ability but they remain highly infectious to sows and gilts. Posterior paralysis is not uncommon along with spondylitis in sucking and weaning pigs.

➤ **PREVENTION**

Herd protection should be considered using the appropriate nosode.

Brucellosis is notifiable in the United Kingdom under the Diseases of Animals Acts and Orders.

Clostridial Infections

Enteritis due to Cl. Perfringens Type C

This fatal necrotic enteritis in susceptible pigs occurs as an acute infection in pigs under seven days old. Affected animals are frequently found dead or suffering from a haemorrhagic diarrhoea. Sub-acute cases may also occur when deaths are less common.

➤ **CLINICAL SIGNS**

Per-acute, acute, sub-acute and chronic forms are recognised. In the per-acute form signs of disease appear one to two days after birth manifested by dysentery. Piglets rapidly become moribund. Sub-normal temperature is usual and the skin may blacken before death. Occasionally one or two pigs may die without showing haemorrhagic diarrhoea.

In the acute form piglets survive slightly longer but invariably die within seven days or so. Diarrhoea sets in containing necrotic material of a brownish colour. Rapid wasting and weakness occurs preceding death.

In the sub-acute form the diarrhoea is non-haemorrhagic but is persistent leading to dehydration and weakness. Necrotic material is also found but the diarrhoea is yellowish in this case. Affected pigs rapidly become emaciated.

In chronic cases pigs develop intermittent diarrhoea over a period up to two weeks. The stools are mucoid and of a yellow-grey colour. General unthriftiness and loss of weight is usual in these cases.

➤ PREVENTION

A multi-valent nosode against the various Clostridial pathogens is available and should be used on a herd basis.

Enteritis due to Clostridium Perfringens Type A

Type A infection has been associated with enteritis in both very young pigs and also in older animals post-weaning. This organism is widespread in nature being regularly found in gut flora and in soils. The majority of young pigs are at risk from this particular infection.

➤ CLINICAL SIGNS

A creamy pasty diarrhoea occurs within 48 hours of birth.

The skin becomes rough while staining from faecal material is seen around the peri-anal area. Temperature usually remains normal, and deaths are infrequent. Diarrhoea may become mucoid and can last up to a week. Recovered pigs remain in poor condition. When weaned pigs become infected the stools are more formed but remain soft. Unthriftiness and loss of condition follow.

Cl. perfringens type A is also capable of causing infection at the site of injections, e.g. iron injections given to treat anaemia. Mortality may be high in these cases. Affected pigs show swelling of the hind limbs (usually involved when iron preparations are employed). These swellings extend along the lower abdomen. The overlying skin is discoloured dark red. The oedema is extensive with an abundance of gas and a brownish red exudate.

➤ **PREVENTION**
A multi-valent nosode should be employed on a herd basis.

Cellulits and Gas Gangrene

Pigs are subject to contamination of wounds by different Clostridial species causing acute inflammation, extensive oedema and local necrosis with production of gas. Inflammation rapidly spreads within infected tissues leading eventually to septicaemia. The organisms concerned are *Cl. septicum, Cl. perfringens A & C, Cl. novyi* and *Cl. chauvoei*. Of these *Cl. septicum* is the one most commonly associated with gas gangrene.

➤ **CLINICAL SIGNS**
The infections run an acute course and can be fatal within 24 hours. Extensive swellings may appear anywhere where a wound has developed. The lower abdominal, inguinal, head and shoulder areas are the commonest sites of infection, extension to adjacent areas taking place in most cases. The skin becomes red and blotchy and develops a purplish colour eventually. Crepitation of the lesions is a constant feature in established infections while pigs are invariably found in lateral recumbency before death.

➤ **PREVENTION**
As in other Clostridial infections the combined nosode should be used.

Blackleg

This particular Clostridial infection is caused by *Cl. chauvoei* but is less common in pigs than in cattle. If pigs do become infected oedema of the sub-mandibular and pharyngeal areas develops.

➤ PREVENTION

As in other Clostridial infections.

Sudden Death Syndrome

This is a description which has been given to animals infected by *Cl. novyi*. As the name suggests sudden un-explained deaths occur in pig units preceded by sub-mandibular swellings, pleural and pericardial effusions.

➤ PREVENTION

As in other Clostridial infections.

Tetanus

This disease is caused by absorption into the system of the toxin of the organism *Cl. tetani* a sporulating anaerobic bacterium which is a common inhabitant of soils especially those which have been heavily manured. Spread of toxin probably through peripheral nerves to the central nervous system eventually affects skeletal muscle producing spasms. Mainly young pigs are affected.

➤ CLINICAL SIGNS

After an incubation period which ranges from several days to several weeks, spasm of voluntary muscles is first seen preceded by a stiffening of the gait. Once infection has been established spread of the disease is rapid. The ears become erect and extension of the tail takes place. Elevation of the head is accompanied by protrusion of the third eyelid. Progression of the disease leads to extension of the limbs which become stiffened and extended posteriorly.

Stimuli such as noise, touch or bright light can exacerbate the spasms. Frothy mucus may be present around the nostrils prior to death.

➤ TREATMENT

1. If the original wound has been of a deep nature by a penetrating object the remedy *LEDUM* is indicated. Suggested potency 6c one dose three times per day for four days.

2. HYPERICUM. This remedy should be used along with the previous one. Suggested potency 1m one dose daily for ten days. The combination of these two remedies has proved successful in preventing the progress of the disease.

3. MAGNESIUM PHOSPHORICUM. This is a useful remedy to control muscular spasms. Suggested potency 30c one dose three times daily for seven days.

4. CURARE. Rigidity and stiffening of muscles are associated with the provings of this remedy. Suggested potency 30c one dose three times daily for seven days.

5. STRYCHNINUM. Extensive arching of the back together with the extension of limbs may be helped by this remedy. Suggested potency 10m one dose twice daily for five days.

6. CL. TETANI NOSODE. This can be combined with any of the suggested remedies using a 30c potency daily for seven days.

➤ **PREVENTION**

As in other Clostridial diseases this could be used on a herd basis.

*B*otulism

This is a disease caused by absorption into the tissues of the toxin produced by the organism *Cl. botulinum* which can exist in decomposing animal or vegetable matter. Infection is by the oral route. Although pigs are less likely to be affected than other species it does occur occasionally. The toxin which is absorbed from the gut affects the neuro-muscular system, death resulting from paralysis of the muscles of respiration.

➤ **CLINICAL SIGNS**

A period ranging from a few hours to a few days passes before clinical signs appear after ingestion of contaminated material. Early signs are loss of tone in voluntary muscles accompanied by weakness, inco-ordination and ataxia. The forelegs usually become affected before the hind ones. All muscles eventually become involved leading to recumbency. Other signs may include dilation of pupils, partial or total loss of sight, involuntary passing of urine and faeces and severe laboured respiration.

➤ **TREATMENT**

If signs of disease can be noted early enough the following remedies may prove helpful, but the successful outcome of any given case will be dependent on the amount of toxin absorbed.

1. NUX VOMICA. This is a useful remedy in the treatment of conditions generally which result from the ingestion of contaminated foods. Suggested potency 1m one dose every hour for four doses.

2. CARBO VEGETABILIS. Like the previous remedy this one also is associated with ingestion of doubtful food, but in this instance fish or fish products are more likely to be incriminated. Suggested potency 200c one dose every hour for four or five doses.

3. LATHYRUS SATIVA. This is a well-proven remedy in the treatment of paralysis of voluntary muscles. Suggested potency 1m one dose three times daily for five days.

4. PLUMBUM. This remedy has a more restricted role concentrating more on single nerves especially radial (fore-legs) and the sciatic (hind-legs). It should therefore be considered as a first choice remedy when fore-leg muscles are involved. Suggested potency 1m one dose twice daily for seven days.

5. BELLADONNA. Dilation of pupils may benefit from this remedy and together with other remedies mentioned above should help prevent deterioration of eyesight.

6. CL. BOTULINUM NOSODE can be used in conjunction with any of the associated remedies using a 30c potency.

7. AGARICUS. Cases of inco-ordination and ataxia should benefit from this remedy. Suggested potency 30c one dose three times daily for five days.

➤ **PREVENTION**
As in other Clostridial diseases.

Swine Erysipelas
This bacterial disease is caused by an organism known as *Erysipelothrix rhusiopathiea*. The condition is widespread in

pig units and is known in most countries of the world. Acute, mild and chronic forms are recognised.

► CLINICAL SIGNS

a) Acute Form. Onset is invariably sudden with a rise in temperature ranging from 104°–108°F. Early bacteraemia leads usually to a more severe septicaemia. If affected pigs survive for a week or two the rise in temperature usually subsides. Diseased pigs separate themselves from the herd and become recumbent. There is stiffness of gait leading to shifting from one leg to the other. Arching of the back is a frequent sign together with the feet tucked under the abdomen. Inactivity of bowels leads to dry stools, although in very young pigs loose motions are sometimes seen. In-pig sows may abort. Reddish or purple spots develop along the ventral surface of the body. In dark-skinned breeds these lesions can be palpated as a guide to their presence.

b) Mild Form. Skin diseases appear as isolated raised usually diamond-shaped patches which become dark and necrotic.

c) Chronic Form. This may follow the acute or mild forms. Arthritis develops, the joints especially of the hind limbs becoming stiff and enlarged. Endocarditis is a common sequel to embarrasment of heart action after exertion. Severe cases develop an inability to put weight on the limbs.

► TREATMENT

1. ACONITUM. If the condition can be detected early enough this remedy is indicated. Suggested potency 10m one dose every hour for four doses.

2. BELLADONNA. This remedy should help control rise in temperature and help prevent bacteraemia developing into more severe complications. Suggested potency 10m one dose every hour for four doses.

3. ECHINACEA. The use of this remedy should help in acute cases and limit the appearance of skin lesions. Suggested potency 6c one dose three times daily for four days.

4. RHUS TOXICODENDRON. Early stiffness of joints will benefit from this remedy and pigs usually show easings of symptoms if made to move. Suggested potency 1m one dose daily for five days.

5. BRYONIA. If pigs resent being made to move and if made to do so immediately assume a recumbent posture this is the indicated remedy. Suggested potency 6c one dose three times daily for five days.

6. ANTHRACINUM. This nosode has given good results in the treatment of mild cases which develop raised dark necrotic lesions. Suggested potency 200c one dose daily for five days.

7. CONVALLARIA. Endocarditis which ultimately affects valvular function of the heart should be helped by this remedy. Suggested potency 3c one dose three times daily for one month. This can be repeated from time to time.

8. OSTEOARTHRITIC NOSODE (OAN). This preparation has reported to be of use in chronic arthritic cases. Suggested potency 200c one dose per week for four weeks.

9. NUX VOMICA. Inactivity of bowel function leading to dry stools should be helped by this remedy. Suggested potency 1m one dose twice daily for five days.

➤ **PREVENTION**
A nosode exists against the causative organism and should be used on a herd basis in 30c potency.

E. Coli Infections

These enteric infections are due to one or other strains of E. coli. This organism is a normal inhabitant of gut flora where its function is to break down food particles and render them suitable for absorption. Disease is likely to occur when under stress, e.g. inclement weather, exposure to prolonged damp conditions, or deprivation of colostrum in the young pig, the E. coli organism assumes pathological significance. E. coli organisms vary considerably in virulence.

Enteric Colibacillosis

This particular condition is associated with diarrhoea which ranges from neo-natal (two to three days after birth) to young pigs up to post-weaning. Haemorrhagic gastro-enteritis develops in older pigs post-weaning.

➤ CLINICAL SIGNS

Diarrhoea varies according to the virulence of the invading organism. Dehydration supervenes due to loss of body fluid. Neo-natal outbreaks may affect whole litters or single pigs. Litters from gilts are more at risk than those from sows. Faeces vary from whitish or creamy to light brown. Vomiting occurs in a proportion of animals accompanied by loss of body weight. The muscles of the abdomen become flaccid. The skin may be bluish or grey extending to the peri-anal area. Diarrhoea is less severe in older pigs. Gastro-enteritis with haemorrhagic stools is confined to older (post-weaning) pigs. Cyanosis of the extremities sometimes develop in these cases together with an occasional brownish stool.

➤ TREATMENT

1. **COLI-GAERTNER.** The combined nosodes of E. coli and Gaertner have given good results in many cases. In practice

it does not seem to matter particularly which strain of *E. coli* is employed but the one which is marketed as *E. COLI* 30c is the one which is recommended (Ainsworths Pharmacy). Suggested potency 30c of the combined nosodes one dose daily for seven days.

2. CHINA OFF. Dehydration and weakness associated with loss of fluid will be helped by this remedy. Suggested potency 6c one dose three times daily for four days.

3. ARSENICUM ALB. Light brown diarrhoea with or without vomiting indicates this remedy. Suggested potency 1m one dose twice daily for five days.

4. LACHESIS. Purplish or dark blue lesions on the skin may be controlled by this remedy especially if they occur over the lower left flank. Suggested potency 30c one dose three times daily for seven days.

➤ **PREVENTION**
E. COLI NOSODE in 30c potency should be used on a herd basis. In-pig sows and gilts will benefit from a twice weekly dose during the last month of pregnancy. This should help limit disease in the new born pig.

*B*owel Oedema

This condition is associated with absorption of toxin produced from various strains of *E. coli*. This is manifested as an enterotoxaemia producing an increase in fluid content of the stomach mucous membrane. The disease usually occurs one to two weeks after weaning in pigs around the ages of four to twelve weeks. Occasionally older animals are affected. Morbidity is low, but deaths can be severe ranging from 50% to 90%. The course of the disease runs from four to fourteen days. One or two affected pigs may recover without any treatment.

> ## CLINICAL SIGNS

Preliminary signs show groups of pigs staggering about and eventually becoming recumbent. Paddling of limbs is a common feature. Loss of appetite and severe diarrhoea of short duration occurs in most cases. Hyperexcitability and nervous twitching occasionally affects a proportion of animals. Eyelids become swollen due to retention of fluid in surrounding tissues. In the later stages of the disease difficult breathing occurs. Temperature is usually normal. Chronic forms may follow the acute unilateral nervous disturbances such as circling movements and lateral deviation of the head developing. Wasting of muscles of limbs may occur. In chronic states subcutaneous oedema is seldom seen.

> ## TREATMENT

1. AGARICUS. This remedy is a most useful one to treat conditions characterised by staggering and ataxia. Suggested potency 30c one dose three times daily for six days.

2. ARSENICUM ALB. Diarrhoea should be helped by this remedy especially if stools contain flecks of blood. Suggested potency 1m one dose twice daily for five days.

3. PHOSPHORUS. Excitability, vomiting and nervous twitchings should benefit from this remedy. Suggested potency 200c one dose daily for five days.

4. APIS MEL. Subcutaneous oedema is associated with this remedy. Suggested potency 30c one dose three times daily for seven days.

5. CICUTA VIROSA. This is a most useful remedy to control nervous symptoms such as circling movements and lateral deviation of the head. Suggested potency 30c one dose three times daily for seven days.

6. E. COLI. The nosode in 30c potency could be used in conjunction with any indicated remedy giving one dose daily for seven days.

➤ PREVENTION
E. coli nosode should be used on a herd basis. If the commercial one proves to be unsuitable a fresh nosode could be used using any affected discharge or blood as the basis for preparation.

E. Coli Mastitis

This condition is also known as Coliform Mastitis and also as Puerperal Mastitis. It is associated with parturition and infection of the mammary gland at that time leading to loss of milk and systemic involvement. The condition is world-wide in distribution. Mortality among affected sows is low but piglets suffer deaths due to lack of milk and possible infection from their dams. The condition is non-contagious.

➤ CLINICAL SIGNS
Early after farrowing symptoms such as loss of milk associated with a rise in temperature and listlessness appear. Difficult breathing and increased heart rate are typical of systemic involvement. The skin over the mammary area becomes inflamed and congested. The mammary glands become firm and are painful on pressure. The inguinal glands are inflamed. Any secretion from the teats tends to be serous and in severe cases creamy.

► **TREATMENT**

1. PHYTOLACCA. This is a well-proven remedy in the treatment of conditions affecting the mammary glands and should always be considered. Suggested potency 30c one dose three times daily for seven days.

2. BRYONIA. Hardness or firmness of the glands may be helped by this remedy. Suggested potency 30c one dose three times daily for five days.

3. BELLADONNA. Heat in the glands along with systemic involvement suggests this remedy. Suggested potency 30c one dose daily for five days.

4. URTICA URENS. This remedy in high potency 200c–1m has been proved useful in promoting milk supply. Suggested dosage one dose daily for seven days.

5. PYROGEN. If there is a discrepancy between temperature and heart rate in any infectious condition this remedy is indicated. Suggested potency 1m one dose every three hours for four doses.

6. E. COLI. This commercial nosode should be used on a daily basis, giving one dose every four hours for three days. A specific nosode made from any particular case is an option if the commercial one proves unsuccessful.

► **PREVENTION**

A polyvalent E. coli nosode should be considered on a herd basis. This should also be employed in sows giving one dose twice per week for the last four weeks of pregnancy.

Exudate Epidermitis

This disease is associated with infection by *Staphylococcus* species especially strains of *Staph. hyicus*. Piglets are normally infected, the condition leading to dehydration and death: weaned pigs and adults are occasionally affected. Affected piglets can be born from non-immune sows. Both morbidity and mortality are fairly high. High humidity is associated with severe outbreaks.

➤ CLINICAL SIGNS

Piglets around four to six days are usually affected, developing a reddish or coppery skin. Brown scales appear on the groin and axillae which are greasy in texture. The skin is hot and the coat becomes matted. The eyes show involvement in the form of exudates and discharges. Ulcers appear in the mouth. The hooves show separation of horn around the bulbs of the heels. Lack of appetite and dehydration accompany these signs. Yellowish skin is a common feature of milder cases. The skin may appear hairy in some cases. Adult pigs show lesions on the back and flanks while ulceration develops in some outbreaks.

➤ TREATMENT

1. MORGAN-PURE OR MORGAN BACH. Either of these nosodes should be used to begin with. They are well proved in the treatment of skin diseases. Suggested potency 30c one dose daily for seven days.

2. SULPHUR. This remedy usually complements the previous one and can be given as a follow-on remedy. Suggested potency 200c one dose every week for three weeks.

3. GRAPHITES. If lesions are more commonly encountered in the axilla and groin areas this remedy may prove useful more especially if there is an accompanying sticky discharge. Suggested potency 30c one dose three times per day for five days.

4. PULSATILLA. This remedy should be indicated in those conditions affecting the eyes. Suggested potency 30c one dose three times daily for five days.

5. BORAX. Mouth ulcers are associated with this remedy. It has a proven record in this condition. Suggested potency 6c one dose three times daily for seven days.

6. SILICEA. Along with the previous remedy, Silicea could be useful in the treatment of foot conditions affecting the bulbs of the heels. It should help delay or prevent the separation of horn. Suggested potency 200c one dose three times per week for four weeks.

7. CHELIDONIUM. Affected pigs which show yellowish skin, implying liver involvement could be helped by this remedy. Suggested potency 30c one dose three times daily for seven days.

8. THALLIUM ACETAS. This is a useful remedy in degenerative and chronic skin conditions and could prove useful in controlling the hairy skin syndrome which appears in some animals. Suggested potency 30c one dose daily for fourteen days.

➤ **PREVENTION**
Polyvalent Staphylococcus nosodes could be employed on a herd basis.

Infection associated with Haemophilus Parasuis

A condition known as Polyserositis with accompanying arthritis has been known to affect pigs which harbour this particular organism. The name Glassers Disease has also been given to this condition which is distributed world-wide. Outbreaks are normally confined to a single farm, young pigs up to eight weeks being the principal sufferers. In severe infections deaths up to half of any particular herd are possible.

➤ CLINICAL SIGNS

Onset of disease symptoms is sudden and the condition is recognised as per-acute or acute. Pigs in the best condition are more at risk than their less nourished companions. An early rise in temperature is followed by loss of appetite. The skin assumes a reddish-purple colour while oedema is noticed around the eyelids, together with conjunctivitis. Movement brings on symptoms of pain. Arthritis develops in knee and hock joints. Involvement of the central nervous system leads to memingoencephalitis, muscular tremors and inco-ordination. Recumbent animals have difficulty in rising.

➤ TREATMENT

1. ACONITUM. This is the principal remedy to be considered in the early stages as soon as symptoms are noticed. Suggested potency 10m one dose every hour for four doses.

2. LACHESIS. Purplish discolouration of the skin calls for this remedy especially if it affects the lower left hand side of the body. Suggested potency 30c one dose three times daily for four days.

3. APIS MEL. This remedy will help alleviate oedema around the eyelids. Suggested potency 30c one dose three times daily for five days.

4. ARGENTUM NITRICUM. Conjunctivitis should be helped by this remedy. Suggested potency 30c one dose three times daily for five days. Other remedies which could be indicated in this condition are *BROMIUM, BORAX, RHUS TOXICODENDRON* and *SYMPHYTUM*. (See Materia Medica for the main indications for each.)

5. BRYONIA. This remedy is the main one to consider in any condition which is aggravated by movement and is therefore indicated for those animals which show pain on being disturbed. Suggested potency 6c one dose three times daily for seven days.

6. ACIDUM SAL. and **OSTEOARTHRITIS NOSODE** are remedies which may help arthritis while *RUTA* should be considered where the main condition is a polyserositis.

7. BELLADONNA. This remedy is called for when encephalitis develops. Suggested potency 1m one dose twice daily for five days.

8. AGARICUS. Inco-ordination due to spinal meningitis may need this remedy, all four limbs being affected. Suggested potency 30c one dose three times daily for seven days.

9. CONIUM. Recumbent animals which have difficulty in rising should benefit from this remedy. Suggested potency 200c one dose daily for seven days.

➤ **PREVENTION**
Haemophilus Nosode should be effective on a herd basis using a 30c potency.

Leptospirosis

Leptospira organisms are capable of causing disease manifested by reproductive failure in breeding herds. The disease occurs in most countries. Abortions, weak pigs and still-births are all hazards to which pregnant sows are exposed.

79

➤ CLINICAL SIGNS

Acute and chronic forms are recognised. In the former an early bacteraemia occurs, accompanied by a rise in temperature. Lack of appetite is seen in affected animals. Jaundice and haemoglobinuria occur in a proportion of pigs, caused by strains of Leptospira known as *L. icterohaemorrhagica*. These symptoms are often transient and although the condition can be severe this acute form is not often encountered. The chronic form of Leptospirosis is more important from an economic point of view and affects in-pig sows resulting in abortions, still births and weak piglets. Resulting infertility adds to the economic problems which arise.

➤ TREATMENT

1. The early pyrexic and bacteraemic phases call for the use of *ACONITUM*. Suggested potency 10m one dose every hour for four doses.

2. NUX VOMICA. This remedy may help to stimulate appetite using a potency of 6c one dose three times daily for three days.

3. MERCURIUS CORROSIVOS. Toxic jaundice dependent on liver involvement calls for the use of this remedy. Suggested potency 30c one dose three times daily for five days.

4. CHELIDONIUM. This remedy is also useful in liver disturbances resulting in jaundice and haemoglobinuria. Suggested potency 30c one dose three times daily for seven days.

5. In-pig sows will benefit from the remedies *VIBURNUM OPULIS* 30c and *CAULOPHYLLUM* also in 30c. The former should be given early in pregnancy, e.g. one dose three times per week for the first three weeks. The latter remedy should be given during the last month one dose twice weekly for four weeks. Caulophyllum has a proven record in reducing the number of late abortions, still births and weak piglets.

6. SEPIA. Infections resulting in infertility should respond to this remedy. It helps restore tone and function to the entire genital tract, and should be used in a potency of 200c once per week for four weeks.

► **PREVENTION**

Nosodes have been prepared against various strains of Leptospira. A polyvalent nosode or one containing L. icterohaemorrhagica and L. pomona by themselves should be sufficient to provide protection on a herd basis.

Mycoplasma Infections

Various species of Mycoplasma are capable of causing a variety of pathological conditions in pig herds. Probably the most important of these is enzootic pneumonia cause by *M. hyopneumoniae*. Another species *M. hyorhinus* is associated with outbreaks of polyserositis and arthritis in young pigs. *M. hyosynoviae* also causes arthritis but is more commonly seen in older pigs.

Mycoplasma Pneumonia

Also known as Enzootic Pneumonia this condition which is found in most countries is a source of serious economic loss. The causative organism *M. hyopneumoniae* colonises the respiratory tract from which spread to susceptible in-contact animals takes place. Although spread within a herd is extremely common the death rate is relatively low and economic loss arises from a sub–standard level of health.

➤ CLINICAL SIGNS

There is an incubation period of ten to sixteen days. Coughing soon develops which becomes chronic and may last for many months. The intensity of coughing is worse in growing and fattening pigs. There is an accompanying loss of appetite. There may be a rise in temperature during stages of acute coughing. Breathing has been described as laboured or 'thumping'. Severely affected pigs become prostrate with disinclination to move.

➤ TREATMENT

1. ACONITUM. This remedy should be given as early as possible when symptoms first appear. Suggested potency 10m one dose every hour for four doses.

2. There is a wide variety of remedies available for the relief of cough in this disease, e.g. *ANTIMONIUM TARTARICUM, ANTIMONIUM ARSENICOSUM, BRYONIA, AMMONIUM CAUSTICUM, BERYLLIUM, PHOSPHORUS* and *SPONGIA* to mention a few. Reference should be made to the section on Materia Medica for the individual characteristics of each. Potencies of 30c should suffice and given three times per day for seven days.

3. PHOSPHORUS. This is a most important remedy when pneumonia has been well established. Breathing is laboured and the cough is rough and dry. Suggested potency 10m one dose three times daily for three days.

4. BRYONIA. Recumbent animals which are disinclined to move will benefit from this remedy. Suggested potency 6c one dose three times daily for five days.

5. MYCOPLASMA NOSODE. The specific nosode in 30c potency can be employed on a daily basis for ten days together with the appropriate remedy.

➤ **PREVENTION**

M. hyopneumonia in 30c potency should be employed on a herd basis.

Pneumonia associated with Pasteurellosis

This condition is caused by *P. multicoda* which develops after primary infection by mycoplasma organisms and occurs more commonly in intensively reared units with insufficient ventilation. Climatic conditions have little influence on the spread or incidence of disease. Pleurisy is also likely to affect a proportion of pigs and is associated with various strains of *P. multicoda* as also are abscesses in lung tissue. The great majority of normal healthy pigs harbour this organism in their nasal cavities and this determines the way by which infection spreads.

➤ **CLINICAL SIGNS**

Acute, sub-acute and chronic forms are recognised.

The acute form is ushered in with a rise in temperature up to 108°F. Purplish discolouration of the abdominal area is occasionally seen together with severe laboured breathing frequently described as 'thumping'.

In the sub-acute form pleurisy develops from the acute stage. Coughing is frequent. Abdominal breathing is seen due probably to pain over the pleural area which restricts proper inspiration. There is loss of weight with a tendency for affected animals to lie on the affected side.

The chronic form is the one most commonly encountered and follows on from the previous stages. Coughing is infrequent and temperature remains normal.

Growing or fattening pigs are most likely to show symptoms.

➤ **TREATMENT**
1. **ACONITUM.** This remedy is indicated in the early stages of the acute form. Suggested potency 10m one dose every hour for four doses.

2. **LACHESIS.** This will be helpful in controlling the purplish discolouration over the abdominal area. Suggested potency 30c one dose three times daily for four days.

3. **PHOSPHORUS.** Laboured (thumping) breathing calls for this remedy. Suggested potency 10m one dose three times per day for two days.

4. **BRYONIA.** This is the main remedy to consider in the treatment of sub-acute conditions showing pleuritic symptoms. Suggested potency 30c one dose three times per day for four days.

5. **ANTIMONIUM TARTARICUM, ANTIMONIUM ARSENICOSUM, AMMONIUM CARB.** and **BERYLLIUM** are remedies which could be indicated to control coughing in chronic cases. (See chapter on Materia Medica for individual indications.)

➤ **PREVENTION**
Pasteurella nosode should be employed on a herd basis using a 30c potency. It is also good practice to treat in-pig sows during the last month of pregnancy giving the nosode three times per week. This should provide some protection via the placenta.

Proliferative Enteropathies of Pigs

These encompass various conditions characterised by thickening of the mucous membranes of the small and less frequently the large intestine. Various names have been assigned to these changes viz. Intestinal Adenomatosis, Necrotic Enteritis, Regional Ileitis and Proliferative Haemorrhagic Enteropathy.

➤ ETIOLOGY

Various species of *CAMPYLOBACTER* bacteria are thought to be implicated.

➤ CLINICAL SIGNS

Pigs at post-weaning stage (around sixteen to twenty weeks of age) are most likely to be affected. In adenomatosis loss of appetite leading to interference with growth, although these signs are not always sufficiently pronounced. There is a general look of dullness and apathy among affected pigs. Diarrhoea is variable but may be more pronounced in older (fattening) pigs, along with loss of appetite. In necrotic and ileitis cases persistent scouring is the rule which may lead to intestinal ulceration and peritonitis. Proliferative haemorrhagic enteropathy shows as an acute haemorrhagic anaemia affecting young adults. Loose black faeces follow in established cases. Death may occur without intestinal symptoms developing, anaemia being the only sign. In-pig sows may abort. Recovery from uncomplicated adenomatosis is not uncommon.

➤ TREATMENT

1. **NUX VOMICA.** This is a remedy which may prove useful in promoting appetite. Suggested potency 1m one dose three times daily for four days.

2. ACIDUM NITRICUM. Intestinal ulceration is a suitable condition for the employment of this remedy and necrotic and ileitis forms will benefit. Suggested potency 200c one dose daily for seven days.

3. CANTHARIS. Cases which progress to peritonitis call for this remedy. The abdomen becomes hard and affected animals resent pressure over this area. Suggested potency 10m one dose three times daily for two days.

4. PHOSPHORUS. This is a remedy which may help less acute cases of haemorrhagic anaemia. Suggested potency 200c one dose three times per week for three weeks.

5. ARSENICUM ALBUM. This remedy should also be considered in those cases which develop black motions. Suggested potency 1m one dose daily for ten days.

6. SILICEA. The basic thickening of the intestinal mucous membranes may respond to this remedy as it has a proven record in the treatment of such conditions. Suggested potency 200c one dose three times per week for four weeks.

7. CAULOPHYLLUM. In-pig sows as in other conditions will benefit from this remedy and help reduce the tendency to abortions. Suggested potency 30c one dose twice weekly for four weeks.

➤ **PREVENTION**
A polyvalent nosode comprising various strains of Campylo bacter should be employed on a herd basis using a potency of 30c.

Salmonellosis

Weaned pigs are the chief group to suffer from infection by Salmonella species. These particular infections are important both from an economic and public health point of view. Recovered animals remain carriers.

➤ ETIOLOGY

There are two main organisms concerned, viz. *S. cholerae suis* and *S. typhinurium*, the former being the more important.

➤ CLINICAL SIGNS

Infection by these bacteria can cause a variety of clinical conditions and symptoms ranging from septicaemia, colitis and pneumonia. Less commonly meningitis, encephalitis and abortion are encountered. Weaned pigs less than five months old are at risk from the septicaemic form although older pigs can also be affected but less commonly. Pigs show a disinclination to move and the appetite is lost. Temperature may rise to 107°F. A moist cough develops and purple discolouration is seen on the extremities and abdomen. Yellow faeces show after about four days, and death rate is high.

The enterocolic (colitis) form is seen most frequently in pigs from weaning to four months of age and acute and chronic forms are recognised, *S. typhinurium* being the commoner organism involved. The faeces are watery and yellow and the diarrhoea may last up to seven days. Relapses are common in the more chronic form with occasional blood-stained stools. Dehydration is variable dependent on the severity of the diarrhoea. Deaths are less common in this form and are due to loss of body fluid over a period of time.

➤ TREATMENT

1. ACONITUM. As in other acute infections this remedy should be given as early as possible. Suggested potency 10m one dose every hour for four doses.

2. PYROGEN. This is a most useful remedy to control septicaemia, the keynote symptom being a discrepancy between pulse and temperature. Suggested potency 1m one dose three times per day for two days.

3. NUX VOMICA. Inappetance calls for this remedy. Suggested potency 1m one dose three times daily for two days.

4. LACHESIS. Purplish discolouration of extremities and abdomen call for this remedy. Suggested potency 30c one dose three times daily for three days.

5. CAMPHORA, CHINA OFFICINALIS, VERATRUM ALBUM and **ALOE** are all remedies which could be indicated in enterocolic cases. (See chapter on Materia Medica for the indications for each: 30c potencies three times daily for seven days may be needed.)

➤ PREVENTION

A combined nosode against the two organisms is called for on a preventive basis, using a 30c potency. This could also be used in treatment combined with any appropriate remedy, one dose daily for ten days.

Diarrhoea due to Spirochaetal Organisms

Colitis affecting weaned pigs is associated with infection by these organisms, various species being incriminated. The disease symptoms which they set up are less severe than in the case of Swine Dysentery. Weaned pigs up to adult status are the group most commonly affected, and carrier animals may follow in some cases. The condition is rare in adults.

➤ CLINICAL SIGNS

There is an incubative period of six to fourteen days. Early signs are hollowness along the flanks accompanied by humped appearance of the back. Oral infection is followed by colonisation of the mucosa of the lower bowel within three to seven days which leads to pasty soft faeces producing staining around the anus. Although appetite is usually maintained condition is lost. Feverish symptoms are invariably absent. Occasionally the faeces are blood-stained.

➤ TREATMENT

1. ACIDUM NITRICUM. This remedy has a proven record in the treatment of colitis and associated conditions affecting the lower bowel. Suggested potency 200c one dose three times per week for three weeks.

2. IRIS VERSICOLOR. Light coloured pasty faeces should respond to treatment by this remedy. It has a marked action on the intestinal tract in general. Suggested potency 30c one dose three times daily for seven days.

3. ALOE. This remedy is also extremely useful in the treatment of colitis and is indicated when animals seek to drink a lot. Stools may be blood-stained accompanied by straining. Suggested potency 30c one dose three times daily for five days.

4. DULCAMARA. Vomiting may be associated with this remedy and infections are worse in autumn where warm days may be followed by cool nights. Faeces may be greenish-tinged if this remedy is indicated. Suggested potency 200c one dose three times per week for three weeks.

5. IODUM. As in the remedy Iris faeces tend to be light coloured. When Iodum is indicated the appetite is maintained and may indeed be excessive. Loss of condition is the rule. Suggested potency 30c one dose daily for fourteen days.

➤ **PREVENTION**

A nosode made from any affected material could be used on a herd basis.

Swine Dysentery

Also known as Vibrionic Dysentery this is a severe muco-haemorrhagic disease affecting mainly growing pigs. It is caused by a spirochaetal organism called *Serpulino* (formerly Treponema) *hyodysenteriae*. The disease is world-wide in distribution.

➤ **CLINICAL SIGNS**

In all cases diarrhoea occurs but this varies according to the virulence of the infection. Rise in temperature is slight. The faeces are at first soft and of a yellow-grey colour. Mucous blood-stained stools follow after a few days. The back becomes arched and there are signs of abdominal pain. Thirst and dehydration accompany emaciation in established cases. Chronic infections lead to dark blood-stained scouring.

➤ **TREATMENT**

1. ACONITUM. If the early pyrexia can be noted in time this remedy will help. Suggested potency 10m one dose every hour for four doses.

2. IRIS VERSICOLOR. Early soft faeces call for this remedy. There is usually tenderness over the region of the liver. Suggested potency 30c one dose three times daily for seven days.

3. COLOCYNTHIS. Arching of the back accompanying abdominal pain may be relieved by this remedy. Suggested potency 1m one dose twice daily for five days.

4. PHOSPHORUS. Animals which exhibit thirst and early blood-flecked stools may be helped by this remedy. Vomiting is occasionally present. Suggested potency 30c one dose three times daily for five days.

5. ARSENICUM ALBUM. This is probably the most important remedy to consider in the more established or chronic forms of the disease, most symptoms of which correspond to provings of this remedy. Suggested potency 1m one dose daily for ten days.

➤ **PREVENTION**
A nosode has been prepared against this disease and can be used both prophylactically and therapeutically, in the latter case along with selected remedies.

Diseases associated with Streptococcal Organisms

Young pigs particularly can be affected by these bacteria causing a variety of conditions ranging from meningitis and arthritis to septicaemic complications of various kinds. Infection is usally introduced to susceptible animals by carrier pigs which may be clinically healthy. Streptococcal bacteria are frequently found to inhabit the tonsils and nasal cavities. Diseases caused by these organisms are more likely to be found in herds which follow an intensive and confined system of management. *S. suis* is the main streptococcal organism associated with disease.

➤ CLINICAL SIGNS

Generally streptococcal infections are associated with a variety of conditions ranging from per-acute cases to sudden death, and in less acute cases to meningitis, anorexia, depression, reddening of skin and feverish states. Inco-ordination leading to paralysis is sometimes seen, preceded by paddling movements, muscle tremors and extreme arching of the back with extension of limbs. Blindness and convulsions occur in other cases. Lameness due to a suppurative arthritis is seen in other outbreaks.

➤ TREATMENT

1. ACONITUM. As in other acute infections this remedy is indicated in the early stages of any attack. Suggested potency 10m one dose every hour for four doses.

2. BELLADONNA, CICUTA VIROSA, CUPRUM METALLICUM, PLUMBUM and **AGARICUS** are remedies which could be indicated for animals which show symptoms of involvement of the central nervous system. Reference should be made to the section on Materia Medica to determine the individual characteristics of each. Suggested potency 30c in each case three times daily for ten days.

3. RHUS TOXICODENDRON. This remedy may help those cases showing reddening of the skin along with early arthritis. Suggested potency 1m one dose daily for fourteen days.

4. CONIUM. This remedy is indicated in those cases which show paddling movements leading to paralysis. Suggested potency 30c–200c–1m. The 30c potency should be given daily for fourteen days followed by 200c potency one dose three times per week for four weeks also for 1m to follow after the 200c.

5. STRYCHNINUM. Extreme arching of the back with extension of limbs calls for this remedy. Suggested potency 1m one dose three times per week for three weeks.

6. SILICEA. The suppuration associated with arthritis should be helped by this remedy. Suggested potency 200c one dose three times per week for four weeks.

7. STREPTOCOCCAL NOSODES. A polyvalent Streptococcal nosode in 30c potency could be used daily for seven days combined with selected remedies.

➤ **PREVENTION**
The same nosode could be used on a herd basis. Also it should be given to in-pig sows during the last four weeks of pregnancy twice per week.

Streptococcal Lymphadenitis

This particular infection is associated with the production of abscesses which develop under the jaws and along the neck. A specific type of streptococcus named *S. porcinus* is thought to be the cause. Carrier animals harbour the organisms in their tonsils. Shedding of organisms occurs via food, water and soil contamination, and also in faeces. Pigs from weaning to marketing are normally affected; also occasionally in sucklers and adults. Infection occurs via the mucous membrane of the pharynx. Abscesses may also occur elsewhere.

➤ **CLINICAL SIGNS**

Abscesses develop in the lymph glands of the neck and throat. A rise in temperature may persist for seven days, followed by loss of appetite, mild diarrhoea and listlessness.

➤ **TREATMENT**

1. **ACONITUM.** Early rise in temperature calls for this remedy. Suggested potency 10m one dose every hour for four doses.

2. **HEPAR SULPH.** This is a well proven remedy in the treatment of septic conditions. The main indication for this remedy is extreme sensitivity to pain. Suggested potency 30c one dose three times daily for five days.

3. **CALC. FLUOR.** This remedy is a useful one for the treatment of infections of glands in particular. It is a most useful tissue remedy and should help restore normal function of the glands. Suggested potency 30c one dose twice daily for fourteen days.

4. **SILICEA.** Well established or so-called chronic cases may benefit from this remedy. Suggested potency 200c one dose three times per week for three weeks.

5. **GAERTNER.** This bowel nosode may help along with selected remedies. It has a beneficial action on the bowel flora and should help in those cases showing mild diarrhoea. Suggested potency 30c one dose daily for seven days.

➤ **PREVENTION**

A nosode developed for the particular organism could be used on a herd basis to prevent infection becoming established in the herd.

Other conditions associated with Streptococcal infections

in pigs and which assume economic importance are septi-caemic complications, arthritis and endocarditis caused mainly by S. *equisimilis*. Skin lesions, tonsillar tissue and the umbilicus are the chief areas which afford entry to the blood-stream: from there infection settles in the joints, the lining of the heart and occasionally in the central nervous system causing meningitis.

➤ CLINICAL SIGNS

Young pigs up to three weeks old are usually affected. Lameness associated with arthritis is an early sign. Temperature is slightly raised. Loss of appetite accompanies a dry harsh coat. Oedema appears around joints as an accompaniment to septic arthritis. A swollen umbilicus is often seen in these cases. Endocarditis produces a picture of prostration with reddening and cyanosis of skin extremities due to valvular incompetence, mainly left-sided.

➤ TREATMENT

1. RHUS TOXICODENDRON. This is a useful remedy in early arthritis cases and should help prevent more serious complications. Suggested potency 1m one dose daily for fourteen days.

2. APIS MEL. The oedema which surrounds joints calls for this remedy. Suggested potency 30c one dose three times daily for four days.

3. OSTEOARTHRITIC NOSODE. This has been developed from synovial fluid and has proved to be a useful remedy in some chronic arthritic conditions. It could be combined with other selected remedies. Potency 30c one dose three times per week for four weeks.

4. PYROGEN. Septic states which combine a rise in temperature and a weak thready pulse (or vice versa) will benefit from this remedy. Suggested potency 1m one dose three times daily for three days.

5. STREPTOCOCCUS NOSODE. Either a specific nosode prepared against *S. equisimilis* or a polyvalent one should prove effective in cases showing umbilical infection together with more general involvement. Suggested potency 30c giving one dose daily for seven days.

6. ADONIS VERNALIS. This is a prominent remedy in connection with valvular disease. Urine output is usually increased and contains albumen and casts. Suggested potency 3x one dose three times daily for thirty days.

7. LAUROCERASUS. Cyanosis of the skin is associated with this heart remedy. Suggested potency 3x as for the previous remedy.

➤ PREVENTION
Streptococcus nosode should be used on a herd basis using a 30c potency.

*P*seudomonas Infections
Pseudomonas bacteria, the chief of which is *P. aeruginosa* are occasionally found in the gut flora of pigs from where endotoxins are released into the system causing infections such as cystitis, uro-genital disease and mastitis. Skin affections may result from contamination.

➤ CLINICAL SIGNS
These are extremely variable. Inflammatory lesions affecting different body systems are seen from time to time. Chronic

ill-defined health problems ensue. Lung abscesses develop leading to coughing of purulent sputum. Chronic pneumonias are often associated with these organisms, leading to bronchitis and emaciation. If infection establishes itself in the intestine, the resultant inflammation leads to a watery brownish diarrhoea. Skin lesions are frequently seen, a serous exudate arising from a crusty inflamed surface.

➤ TREATMENT

1. CANTHARIS. This is a principal remedy for the treatment of cystitis. Suggested potency 10m one dose three times daily for three days.

2. BELLADONNA. Inflammatory conditions affecting the mammary glands call for this remedy. The glands feel hot with a shiny surface. Suggested potency 1m one dose every two hours for four doses.

3. PHYTOLACCA. Mastitis which may have been helped by the previous remedy should benefit from this one as a follow-on. It should help prevent abscesses developing. Suggested potency 30c one dose three times daily for five days.

4. KREOSOTUM. This remedy may prove useful in pneumonic cases leading to abscesses with purulent sputum. Suggested potency 200c one dose daily for ten days.

5. ARSENICUM ALBUM. Enteric cases developing watery diarrhoea should benefit from this remedy. Suggested potency 1m three times daily for three days.

6. PYROGEN. Septic states in general may need this remedy when temperature and pulse are in imbalance. Suggested potency 1m one dose three times daily for three days.

7. HEPAR SULPH. Inflamed lesions on the skin leading to serous exudate may need this remedy. Suggested potency 30c three times daily for four days.

➤ PREVENTION
P. aeruginosa nosode 30c should be used on a herd basis.

Infection due to Actinobacillus suis

This bacillus (*A. suis*) has been implicated in septiacemic infections resulting in death mainly in piglets and weaners. The organism lodges in the tonsils and posterior nares of healthy pigs and also in vaginal secretions. Infection probably occurs via the upper respiratory tract and also through skin abrasions and mucous membranes. Pyaemia can follow causing necrotic foci in various parts of the body. Severe infections can result in death within fifteen hours.

➤ CLINICAL SIGNS
The organism is associated with sudden deaths and as such should be viewed with suspicion. Slight pyrexia is first seen in piglets which become ill. Cyanosis of the skin accompanied by petechial haemorrhages also occurs in many outbreaks. Necrosis of the tip of the tail and ears is preceded by local congestion. Persistent cough and pneumonia occur in pigs at weaning time. Occasionally meningitis has been reported in older animals while sows have developed metritis.

➤ TREATMENT
1. ACONITUM. This is the usual remedy to be considered in the early pyrexic state. Suggested potency 10m one dose every hour for four doses.

2. LACHESIS. This remedy should help those cases which

show cyanosis. Suggested potency 30c one dose three times daily for four days.

3. PHOSPHORUS. Petechial haemorrhages are associated with this remedy. Suggested potency 200c one dose daily for five days.

4. SECALE. Congestion and necrosis of extremities call for this remedy. Suggested potency 200c one dose three times per week for three weeks.

5. BRYONIA, PHOSPHORUS, ANTIMONIUM ARSENICOSUM, LYCOPODIUM, TUBERCULINUM AVIARE and **ANTIMONIUM TARTARICUM** are all remedies which could be indicated for the treatment of pneumonic cases. (See chapter on Materia Medica for their individual characteristics.)

6. PYROGEN. Mastitis in sows could be helped by this remedy. Suggested potency 1m one dose three times daily for four days.

➤ PREVENTION
A nosode prepared from infected material could form the basis for herd prevention.

Staphylococcal Infections

Staphylococcal organisms are widespread in distribution and can affect pigs of all ages causing a variety of clinical conditions. The chief bacterium is *S. aureus* although *S. hyicus* is also important. *S. aureus* can be recovered from various body systems such as respiratory and uro-genital. Infection can result from contamination or by oral means. Local infections of mammary glands, umbilicus and skin are common. Spread to other tissue via the blood-stream can lead to multiple abscesses developing. When bone structures are involved osteomyelitis may result. Pyaemia can lead to septic arthritis.

➤ CLINICAL SIGNS

These are variable. Neonatal septicaemia can lead to the development of abscesses around the umbilicus and joints. Staphylococci are also associated with foot lesions leading to arthritis of small joints. Septic involvement of the coronary band may follow. A guiding symptom of *S. aureus* infection is the presence of a creamy blood-stained pus.

➤ TREATMENT

1. HEPAR SULPH. Early septicaemic cases may be helped by this remedy and it should help prevent further spread. Suggested potency 1m one dose three times daily for three days.

2. TARENTULA CUBENSIS. This is a useful remedy to treat abscesses and boils which may appear in different areas, e.g. the umbilicus and around joints. Suggested potency 30c one dose three times daily for five days.

3. CAULOPHYLLUM, ACTAEA RACEMOSA, ACIDUM SALICYLIC and **LITHIUM CARBONICUM** are remedies which could in their own way be relevant in the treatment of small joint arthritis (see Materia Medica).

4. SILICEA. Chronic septic states including infection of the coronary band should benefit from this remedy. Suggested potency 200c one dose three times per week for four weeks.

5. STAPHYLOCCUS NOSODE. A combined nosode is always indicated in treatment combined with other remedies. Suggested potency 30c one dose daily for seven days.

> **PREVENTION**

The same nosodes are available for protection.

Corynebacterium Infection

This is associated with an organism known as *C. suis* and has been implicated in infections of the urinary tract such as cystitis and pyelonephritis. The organism is found in the prepuce of male pigs. Sows and gilts suffer from urinary infections. Spread to the kidney pelvis results from an ascending infection from the bladder. The disease in sows frequently follows mating or parturition.

> **CLINICAL SIGNS**

Blood in urine is a usual sign in acute infections. Loss of weight occurs. Catarrhal involvement of mucous membranes of urethra bladder and ureters leads on to a purulent and/or haemorrhagic discharge.

> **TREATMENT**

1. **BERBERIS VULGARIS.** This is a prominent remedy in the control of haematuria and kidney/bladder conditions generally. Suggested potency 30c one dose three times daily for five days.

2. **HYDRASTIS.** Catarrhal conditions of mucous membranes should be treated by this remedy. Suggested potency 30c one dose three times daily for six days.

3. **PAREIRA.** Severe straining with discharge of mucus from the urethra may indicate this remedy. Suggested potency 6c one dose three times daily for seven days.

4. **CHIMAPHILLA UMBELLATA.** Urine is passed with straining and contains more purulent material than blood. The

urine is dark green and strong-smelling. Suggested potency 6c one dose three times daily for six days.

5. UVA URSI. signs of discomfort accompany the passage of greenish slimy urine containing blood and purulent material. Suggested potency 6c one dose three times daily for five days.

➤ PREVENTION
Corynebacterium nosodes are available for protection.

Infection due to Actinomyces pyogenes
This relates to conditions of a suppurative nature in pigs and is widespread occurring in various countries. Infection can take many and varied forms, mastitis, pneumonia and arthritis being some of the more common, along with abscesses of differing degrees of severity.

➤ CLINICAL SIGNS
Paraplegia or paralysis due to osteomyelitis. Cellulitis around joints occurs, leading to arthritis. The colour of the pus is significant viz. greenish.

➤ TREATMENT
1. CONIUM. This is a useful remedy to consider in the treatment of paraplegic conditions provided the nerves are not completely dead. Different potencies ranging from 30c up to 10m may be needed, three times per day for the former for five days and three times per week for four weeks for the latter.

2. PHYTOLACCA. This is a useful remedy to consider in mastitis. Suggested potency 30c one dose three times daily for six days.

3. ANTIMONIUM TARTARICUM. Pneumonic conditions may respond to this remedy. Suggested potency 30c three times daily for seven days. Other remedies which could prove helpful are *LYCOPODIUM* and *BRYONIA* (see Materia Medica).

4. ACIDUM SALICYLIC. This is a remedy which should be considered in arthritis. Suggested potency 200c one dose three times per week for four weeks.

5. MERCURIUS SOL. The greenish nature of the pus is a keynote for this remedy and may be helpful in the treatment of cellulitus and osteomyelitis. Suggested potency 30c one dose three times daily for seven days.

➤ **PREVENTION**
Actinomyces nosode should be considered.

CHAPTER NINE

OTHER *Specific Conditions*

Eperythrozoonosis

This condition is caused by a rickettsial organism named *E. suis*. It causes illness among feeder pigs characterised by fever and jaundice. In-pig sows have also been reported to be affected. Subclinical and carrier states exist. Immunity to this infection may be short lived as any condition leading to stress can reactivate the infection.

➤ CLINICAL SIGNS

Young pigs up to around one week exhibit pale skin and jaundice. In mild cases recovery may set in after a week or two. Growth in feeder pigs is retarded but jaundice in this group is uncommon. In-pig sows exhibit both acute and chronic infections. Loss of appetite is followed by oedema of mammary and vulval areas. Milk secretion tends to dry up and new-born piglets are neglected by the sow. Mild cases may recover after farrowing. There is a decrease in conception rates at the first oestrus after farrowing. Chronic states show jaundice and weakness with anaemic or pale skin and mucous membranes. Delayed oestrus is a common sequel along with a permanent loss of condition.

➤ TREATMENT

1. CHELIDONIUM. This is one of the main remedies to be considered in the control of jaundice which is merely a symptom that liver function is sub-normal. Suggested potency 30c one dose three times daily for seven days.

2. ARSENICUM ALB. This remedy has proved useful in the treatment of anaemic conditions. Suggested potency 1m one dose daily for fourteen days.

3. APIS MEL. Oedematous conditions of the mammary gland and vulva should benefit from this remedy. Suggested potency 200c one dose daily for seven days.

4. SEPIA. If sows show indifference to their young this well-proven remedy may help. Suggested potency 200c one dose daily for three days. This remedy will also prove helpful in treating any sows which show lack of oestrus.

5. URTICA URENS. This remedy in high potency 200c–1m is useful in the treatment of sows which suffer loss of milk at farrowing time. One dose should be given daily for five days.

➤ **PREVENTION**
No vaccines (or nosodes) exist for the prevention of this disease, but it should be possible to prepare a nosode from blood taken from an infected case in the early feverish phase.

Chlamydia Infection

Chlamydial organisms can affect many species and the main one which concerns pig producers is *C. pisittaci*, and although associated more with avian infection occasionally produces disease in mammalian species. A variety of conditions can cause infection such as pneumonia, pleurisy, pericarditis, arthritis, orchitis and uterine complications which can result in abortion. Pigs can become infected through contact with diseased birds or their droppings. Genital tract infection can result from coitus.

➤ CLINICAL SIGNS

There is an incubation period of three to eleven days. A rise in temperature accompanies a loss of appetite. Pneumonia is a frequent complication and is usually associated with pleurisy and pericarditis. Conjunctivitis develops in some animals. Arthritis and nervous signs are additional complications. Piglets become unsteady with a staggering gait. Disturbances of reproduction result in abortions, weak and dead piglets. In boars testicular swellings and urethritis are seen.

➤ TREATMENT

1. ACONITUM. This remedy is indicated in the early pyrexic state. Suggested potency 10m one dose every hour for four doses.

2. NUX VOMICA. Loss of appetite will be helped by this remedy. Suggested potency 1m one dose twice daily for five days.

3. PHOSPHORUS. If this remedy is given early in pneumonic cases it should help prevent progression to more serious disease. Suggested potency 10m one dose every two hours for four doses.

4. BRYONIA. This is the main remedy in cases of pleurisy. Affected animals are disinclined to move and tend to lie on the affected side. This remedy will also help relieve pericarditis. Suggested potency 30c three times daily for four days.

5. ACID SALICYLIC. This is a useful remedy for the treatment of arthritic cases. Suggested potency 200c one dose three times per week for four weeks.

6. AGARICUS. Meningitis leading to nervous signs such as staggering and weak gait may benefit from this remedy. Suggested potency 30c one dose three times daily for seven days.

7. CAULOPHYLLUM. Reproductive disorders in sows and gilts call for this remedy. It should help limit abortions and weak piglets etc. Suggested potency 30c one dose three times per week for four weeks early in the infection.

8. HEPAR SULPH. Testicular infection and urethritis in boars are likely to improve with this remedy. Suggested potency 30c one dose three times daily for seven days.

➤ **PREVENTION**
Chlamydia nosodes are available to be used on a herd basis.

Fungus Infections

Candida albicans – a yeast – has been recovered from the throat, alimentary tract and urogenital system of pigs. This can arise when inflammation of these structures has followed the prolonged use of antibiotics. Candida is spread in faeces and exhalations and is found in weakened skin and mucous surfaces.

➤ **CLINICAL SIGNS**
Chronic gastro-enteritis has been associated with this organism also causing cutaneous and pharyngeal ulcerations. Dullness, loss of appetite and vomiting are accompanying signs. Diarrhoea of a grey-black colour also affects a proportion of animals. This tends to become chronic. Circular pale lesions often appear on the tongue and hard palate. Skin lesions yield a moist exudate together with loss of hair and thickening of skin.

➤ TREATMENT

1. ARSENICUM ALBUM. This is a most useful remedy for controlling gasto-enteritis with or without vomiting. Suggested potency 1m one dose three times daily for four days.

2. ACIDUM NITRICUM. Ulcerations around the mouth and pharyngeal areas should benefit from this remedy. Suggested potency 200c one dose three times per week for two weeks.

3. BORAX. This is also a useful remedy when ulceration affects the mucous membranes of the mouth and pharynx. An indication for its use is excessive salivation and dis-inclination to move in a downward direction. Suggested potency 6c one dose three times daily for seven days.

4. GRAPHITES. Skin lesions yielding a moist exudate may need this remedy. Suggested potency 30c one dose three times daily for five days.

➤ PREVENTION

A candida nosode has been prepared and should be considered to give protection on a herd basis using a 30c potency.

Coccidiosis

The name *coccidia* is reserved for a group of protozoal parasites which cause disease in birds and various mammalian species. Eimeria, Isospora and Cryptosporidium are names given to various types, *Isospora suis* being the one incriminated in disease in pigs. It affects neo-natal piglets and occurs in most countries.

➤ CLINICAL SIGNS

These appear between seven and fourteen days after ingestion of the parasite. The first sign is a greyish-yellow diarrhoea which becomes more fluid as the disease progresses.
The faeces have a sour smell. Infestation can be high in pig
units but deaths are not high. Loss of weight and dehydration are usual signs. When deaths occur they are frequently
associated with secondary infections. Older pigs are less
likely to be affected.

➤ TREATMENT

1. IPECACUANHA. The diarrhoea associated with this
particular condition calls for this remedy to be considered
because of its alkaloid content which has proved effective in
amoebic dysentery. Suggested potency 6c one dose three
times daily for ten days.

2. MERCURIUS CORROSIVUS. This is a well proven remedy
in dysenteric conditions accompanied by straining and the
passage of mucus stools especially in the period from sunset
to sunrise. Suggested potency 200c one dose daily for seven
days.

3. SYCOTIC CO. This is a bowel nosode and is a useful
adjunct accompanying the other remedies. It is useful in the
treatment of enteric catarrhal conditions generally.
Suggested potency 6c one dose three times per day for six
days.

➤ PREVENTION

Protozoal diseases are difficult to prevent in contrast to
bacterial or viral diseases but the bowel nosode *SYCOTIC
CO* should be tried on a herd basis. In this connection a
potency of 30c should be employed.

The protozoal organism *CRYPTOSPORIDIUM PARVUM* can also cause disease in pigs causing a non-haemorrhagic diarrhoea affecting piglets of six to twelve weeks. *IPECACUANHA* as above could be helpful in treatment.

Toxoplasmosis

A protozoal parasite named *Toxoplasma gondii* is responsible for disease in various species. Infection takes place from ingestion of oocysts. Pigs become infected from contamination via cat faeces which is the species responsible for spread. The specific organism is related to the coccidia family.

➤ CLINICAL SIGNS

Symptoms of disease in pigs are not always apparent at first glance. Diarrhoea may occur in severe infestations. Sows may abort in some outbreaks.

➤ TREATMENT

This depends on observations of pigs and how any individual animal responds to the trouble. Diarrhoea could be controlled by remedies such as *IPECACUANHA*, *MERCURIUS CORROSIVUS*, *SYCOTIC CO.* and *ACIDUM NITRICUM*. (See chapter on Materia Medica.)

External Parasites

The most important of these in pigs is SARCOPTIC MANGE caused by the parasite *S. scabei (var. suis)*. The condition is important from an economic point of view because of inability of affected pigs to settle properly due to excessive itching. The condition is widespread in distribution.

➤ **CLINICAL SIGNS**

The most obvious sign is itching which leads to a chronic skin condition affecting a few or many animals. The main symptoms are seen around six weeks. Encrustations on the ear are early signs leading to the development of plaques. The skin over the rump becomes reddened, and this extends forward to the flank and abdomen. Scabs eventually form.

➤ **TREATMENT**

As an accompaniment to external dressings which are essential, the remedy *SULPHUR* should be used in 200c potency one dose every week for three weeks. *PETROLEUM* 30c may be needed to control the reddened patches which develop and also any scarring or thickening which may arise.

Worming

The question of worming in the domesticated animal by homoeopathy is a contentious one inasmuch as homoeopathic remedies do not actually act as Vermicides. The theory behind homoeopathic worming is based on the belief that these remedies, while not actually killing worms, will render the stomach and intestinal tract unsuitable for the establishment or development of worms. This has proved successful in horses and cattle so it is reasonable to assume that the same procedure will be of benefit in pig practice.

It is the author's practice to advise farmers first to employ a conventional wormer and to follow this with a homoeopathic remedy. As the main worm infestations in pigs are due to various species of round worm, the following remedies should be considered: *KAMALA*, *GRANATUM*,

CHENOPODIUM and TEUCRIUM used in 30c potency. The approach which the author advises is to dissolve ten powders of the appropriate remedy in 500ml distilled water. From this stock solution 20ml should be added to the feed daily for four weeks. This regime can be repeated after an interval of two weeks. Of the remedies mentioned KAMALA has proved the most successful for general use in older animals while CHENOPODIUM acts better in young stock.

Nosodes

Reference to nosodes and oral vaccines has already been made in the preface of this book and it is only necessary to add that all disease products are rendered innocuous after the third centesimal potency which is equivalent to a strength or dilution of 1/000/000. They are usually used in 6c or 30c.

BACILLINUM

This is one of the tuberculosis nosodes and is mainly used in the treatment of ringworm and similar skin conditions.

E. COLI NOSODE

This is prepared from various strains of E. coli and is used in pig practice to help control Coliform Mastitis and Colibaccillosis of young piglets.

STREPTOCOCCUS NOSODE

Prepared from various strains of haemolytic Streptococci. It is used as a supplementary remedy in various infections associated with these bacteria.

SALMONELLA NOSODE

Prepared from the common Salmonella organisms associated with this disease and used both prophylactically and therapeutically.

SYCOTIC CO.

This is one of a group of nosodes prepared from the non-lactose fermenting baccilli found in the large intestine. Each one is related to certain homoeopathic remedies and used mainly in conjunction with them. This particular nosode is used in coccidiosis in pig practice.

MORGAN

This bowel nosode is associated with inflammatory conditions especially those of the skin.

GAERTNER

Marked emaciation or malnutrition is associated with this nosode. Chronic gastro-enteritis occurs.

DYS. CO.

This nosode is chiefly concerned with the digestive and cardiac systems. Pyloric spasm occurs with retention of digested stomach contents leading to vomiting. There is functional disturbance of the heart's action.

OSTEO-ARTHRITIC NOSODE

The ø is prepared from fluid taken from an osteo-arthritis joint and dissolved in alcohol. It is a remedy which has a place in the treatment of degenerative joint conditions and could prove useful in chronic Swine Erysipelas along with selected remedies.

CHAPTER TEN

MATERIA *Medica*

ACIDUM NITRICUM. Potencies are prepared from a solution in distilled water. This acid particularly affects body outlets where skin and mucous membranes meet. It produces ulceration and blisters in the mouth and causes offensive discharges. The ulceration may also affect mucous membranes elsewhere and it has been of benefit in some forms of colitis.

ACIDUM SALICYLICUM. Trituration of powder and thereafter potentised. This acid has an action on joints producing swellings and in some cases caries of bone. Gastric symptoms, e.g. bleeding are also prominent in its proving. Homoeopathically it is indicated in the treatment of rheumatic and osteo-arthritis conditions and idiopathic gastric bleeding.

ACID SULPHUROUS. Potencies are prepared from solution in water. The respiratory system is affected by this remedy producing coughing and difficulty in breathing.

ACONITUM NAPELLUS. (MONKSHOOD). In the preparation of the ø the entire plant is used as all parts contain the active principle. This plant has an affinity for serous membranes and muscular tissues leading to functional disturbances.

There is sudden involvement and tension in all parts. This remedy should be used in the early stages of all feverish conditions where there is sudden appearance of symptoms which may also show an aggravation when any extreme of temperature takes place. Predisposing factors which may produce a drug picture calling for Aconitum include shock operation and exposure to cold dry winds or dry heat.

ACTAEA RACEMOSA. (SNAKE ROOT). Potencies are prepared from trituration of the resin. This plant resin has a wide range of action on various body systems chief among which are the female genital and articular leading to disturbances of the uterus in particular and small joint arthritis. Muscular pains are evident, affection of cervical vertebrae being evidenced by stiffening of neck muscles.

ADONIS VERNALIS. (PHEASANTS EYE). Potencies are prepared from infusion of the fresh plant. The main action of the remedy which concerns us in veterinary practice is its cardiac action, the heart becoming weak leading to dropsy and scanty output of urine. It is one of the main remedies used in valvular disease and difficult respiration dependent on pulmonary congestion.

AGARICUS MUSCARIUS. (FLY AGARIC). The ø is prepared from the fresh fungus. Muscarin is the best known toxic compound of several which are present in this fungus. Symptoms of poisoning are generally delayed from anything up to twelve hours after ingestion. The main sphere of action is on the central nervous system producing a state of vertigo and delirium followed by sleepiness. There are four recognised stages of brain involvement viz. 1. Slight stimulation. 2. Intoxication. 3. Delirium 4. Depression with soporific tendency. These actions determine its use in certain conditions affecting the central nervous system, e.g. meningitis and ataxia.

ALOE. (SOCOTRINE ALOES). The ø is prepared from a solution in spirit of the gum resin. Where disease and drug symptoms are confused this remedy is useful in restoring physiological equilibrium. Congestion of the portal circulation is the main result of material doses of this substance. It is a useful remedy in colitis showing abdominal flatulence. Straining at stool occurs with jelly-like stools containing mucus.

AMMONIUM CARBONICUM. This salt is used as a solution in distilled water from which the potencies are made. It is primarily used in respiratory affections especially when there is an accompanying swelling of associated lymph glands. Emphysema and pulmonary oedema are thoracic conditions which may be helped by this remedy. It is also useful in digestive upsets.

AMMONIUM CAUSTICUM. Potencies are again prepared from a solution in distilled water. This salt has a similar but more pronounced action on mucous membranes to that of the carbonate producing ulceration on these surfaces. It is also a powerful heart stimulant. Respiratory conditions such as pneumonia with 'thumping' breathing should benefit from its use. There is usually an excess of mucus when this remedy is indicated.

AMYL NITROSUM (NITRITE). Potencies are prepared from solution in water. It is used mainly in chest conditions where a lack of oxygen (air hunger) appears to affect the animal. This is manifested by mouth breathing and increased respirations. The heart action becomes laboured.

ANTHRACINUM. The ø is prepared from affected tissue and dissolved in alcohol. This nosode is indicated in the treatment of eruptive skin diseases which are characterised by reddish or blackened swellings e.g. swine erysipelas. Cellular tissue becomes indurated and swelling of associated lymph glands occurs.

ANTIMONIUM ARSENICOSUM. Potencies are prepared from trituration of the dried salt dissolved in distilled water. This salt possesses a selective action on the lungs especially the left area and is used mainly in the treatment of emphysema and long-standing pneumonias. Coughing if present is worse on eating and the animal prefers to stand rather than lie down.

ANTIMONIUM TARTARICUM. Trituration of the dried salt is the source of the potencies. Respiratory symptoms predominate with the drug, affection being accompanied by the production of excess mucus, although expectoration is difficult. The main action being on the respiratory system we should expect this remedy to be beneficial in conditions such as broncho-pneumonia and pulmonary oedema. Ailments requiring this remedy frequently show an accompanying drowsiness and lack of thirst. In pneumonic states the edges of the eyes may be covered with mucus.

APIS MELLIFICA (BEE VENOM). The ø is prepared from the entire insect and also from the venom diluted with alcohol. The venom of the bee acts on cellular tissue causing oedema and swelling. The production of oedema anywhere in the system may lead to a variety of acute and chronic conditions, We should consider this remedy in conditions showing oedematous swellings. Synovial swellings of joints and respiratory conditions showing an excess of pulmonary oedema call for its use. Animals are invariably thirstless.

ARGENTUM NITRICUM. This remedy is prepared by trituration of the salt dissolved in alcohol or distilled water. It produces inco-ordination of movement causing trembling in various parts. It has an irritant effect on mucous membranes producing a free-flowing muco-purulent discharge. Red blood cells are affected, anaemia being caused by their destruction. Its sphere of action makes it a useful remedy in eye conditions.

ARNICA MONTANA. (LEOPARDS BANE). The ø is prepared from the whole fresh plant. The action of this remedy produces bruising and swelling and should be used in any condition where injuries occur provided the skin is unbroken. It will help control bleeding after surgical interferances.

ARSENICUM ALBUM. This remedy is prepared by trituration and subsequent dilution. It is a deep acting remedy and acts on every tissue and its characteristic symptoms determine its use in many conditions. Discharges are acrid and symptoms are relieved by heat. It is of use in many skin conditions associated with dryness, scaliness and itching. It could be particularly effective in Swine Dysentery. Animals needing this remedy drink small quantities of water frequently.

AURUM METALLICUM. Potencies are prepared by trituration and subsequent dilution in alcohol. This remedy in the crude state produces an action on bone and cartilage causing ulceration and necrosis. It could prove of value in animals affected with Atrophic Rhinitis.

BELLADONNA. (DEADLY NIGHTSHADE). The ø is prepared from the whole plant at flowering. This plant produces a profound action on every part of the central nervous system causing a state of excitement and active congestion. One of the main guiding symptoms in prescribing is the presence of a full bounding pulse in any feverish condition which may or may not accompany excitable states. Another guiding symptom is dilation of pupils.

BERBERIS VULGARIS. (BARBERRY). The ø is prepared from the bark of the root. This plant has an affinity with most tissues. The chief ailments which come within its sphere of action are those connected with the liver and kidneys. Jaundice frequently attends such conditions. Haematuria and cystitis may occur. In all these conditions there is an accompanying sacral weakness and tenderness over the loins.

BORAX. Potencies are prepared from trituration of the salt dissolved in distilled water. This salt produces gastro-intestinal irritation with mouth symptoms of salivation and ulceration: with most complaints there is fear of downward motion.

BROMIUM. Potencies are prepared from solutions in distilled water. This element acts chiefly on the mucous membranes of the respiratory tract especially the upper trachea causing laryngeal spasm. Its indication in respiratory ailments is related to symptoms being aggravated on inspiration. It may be of use also in those conditions which arise from exposure to heat.

BRYONIA ALBA. (WHITE BRYONY). The ø is prepared from the root before flowering takes place. This important plant exerts its main action on epithelial tissues and also on serous and synovial membranes. Some mucous surfaces are also affected producing an inflammatory response resulting in a fibrinous or serous exudate. This in turn leads to dryness of the affected tissue with later effusions into synovial cavities.

Movement of the parts is interfered with and this leads to one of the main indications for its use viz. all symptoms are worse from movement, the animal preferring to lie still. Pressure over any affected area relieves symptoms. This remedy is useful in treating the many respiratory conditions met with especially pleurisy.

CALCAREA FLUORICA. Potencies are prepared from trituration of the salt with subsequent dilution in distilled water. The special sphere of action of this remedy lies in its relation to bone lesions especially exostosis. It also has an action on glandular tissue causing conditions such as lymphadenitis.

CALCAREA PHOSPHORICA. Potencies are prepared from trituration and subsequent dilution. This salt has an affinity with tissues which are concerned with growth and the repair of cells. Brittleness of bone is a common feature. This is a remedy of special value in the treatment of musculo-skeletal disorders of young stock.

CAMPHORA. Potencies are prepared from a solution of the gum in rectified spirit. This substance produces a state of collapse with weakness and failing pulse. There is icy coldness of the entire body. Any form of enteritis showing exhaustion and collapse may require this remedy. It could be indicated in disease caused by Salmonella species.

CANTHARIS. The ø is prepared by trituration of the insect with subsequent dilution in alcohol. The poisonous substance contained in Cantharis (Spanish Fly) attacks particularly the urinary and sexual organs setting up violent inflammation. The skin is also markedly affected, a severe vesicular rash developing with intense itching. This is a valuable remedy in nephritis and cystitis. The urine contains blood as a rule. It could also be indicated in eczemas showing vesicular inflammation.

CARBO VEGETABILIS. Potencies are prepared by trituration and subsequent dilution in alcohol. Various tissues of the body have a marked affinity with this substance. The circulatory system is particularly affected leading to lack of oxygenation. This is a useful remedy in cases of collapse. Pulmonary congestion may benefit from its use. It acts more on the venous than on the arterial circulation.

CAULOPHYLLUM. (BLUE COHOSH). The ø is prepared from trituration of the root dissolved in alcohol. This plant produces an action on the female genital system. Early abortions occur: also retention of afterbirth and mummified foetuses. In potentised form this remedy will relieve labour pains and could be used as an alternative to pituitrin injections in weak labour. This is an important remedy in many pig diseases leading to abortions, still births and mummified foetuses especially in Respiratory and Reproductive Disease (Blue Ear Disease).

CHELIDONIUM. (GREATER CELANDINE). The ø is prepared from the whole plant, fresh at the time of flowering. A specific action on the liver is produced. There is general lethargy and indisposition. The tongue is coated a dirty yellow and signs of jaundice may be seen in other visible mucous membranes. The liver is constantly upset with the production of clay-coloured stools. It should be remembered when dealing with disturbances associated with a sluggish liver action.

CHENOPODIUM. (WORM SEED). The ø is prepared from the root dissolved in alcohol. This is one of the main remedies for use in the treatment and prevention of round worms in young animals (see chapter on worming).

CHIMAPHILLA UMBELLATA. (GROUND HOLLY). The ø is prepared from the fresh plant. The active principle of this plant produces a marked action on the kidneys and genital system of both sexes. The urine is mucoid and blood-stained.

CHINA OFFICINALIS (CINCHONA) QUININE. The ø is prepared from the dried bark dissolved in alcohol. Large doses of this substance produces toxic changes e.g. haemorrhages, fever and diarrhoea. Weakness ensues from loss of body fluid. This remedy should be considered when any animal is suffering from debility or exhaustion after fluid loss, e.g. severe diarrhoea or haemorrhage.

CICUTA VIROSA. (WATER HEMLOCK). The ø is prepared from the fresh root when the plant flowers. This plant exerts its main influence on the central nervous system giving rise to spasmodic affections. The head is turned or twisted to one side. Cerebro-spinal disorder may benefit from its use. The head may bend backwards with the neck curved.

COLOCYNTHIS. (CUCUMBER). The ø is prepared from the fruit. This plant is purgative and causes violent inflammation of the gastro-intestinal tract. Both onset of and relief from symptoms are abrupt. Diarrhoea is yellowish and forcibly expelled. Relief is obtained by movement while aggravation occurs after eating or drinking.

CONIUM MACULATUM. (HEMLOCK). The ø is prepared from the fresh plant. The alkaloid of this plant produces a paralytic action on nerve ganglia especially the motor nerve endings. This leads to stiffness and a paralysis which tends to travel forward or upward. This remedy is of importance in treating paraplegic conditions affecting the hind limbs.

CONVALLARIA. (LILY OF THE VALLEY). The ø is prepared from the fresh plant. The active principle of this plant has the power to increase the quality of the heart's action and this determines its main use as a remedy in congestive heart conditions. It has little action on heart muscle and is used mainly in valvular disease. It could be of value in the cardiac symptoms of Swine Erysipelas.

CROTALUS HORRIDUS. (RATTLESNAKE VENOM). This is the poison of the rattlesnake and potencies are prepared from the venom with lactose and subsequent dilution in alcohol. The marked action of this poison on the vascular system makes it a valuable remedy in the treatment of many low-grade septic states with circulatory involvement, e.g. puerperal fever and wound infections. Septic conditions are accompanied by oozing of blood from any body orifice and are usually attended by jaundice.

CUPRUM METALLICUM. The ø is prepared from trituration of the metal and subsequent dilution. The symptoms produced by this remedy are characterised by violence including paroxysm of cramping muscle pains which follow no particular pattern. Muscles become contracted and show twitching. In the central nervous system fits and convulsions occur and may take an epileptiform nature.

CURARE. (ARROW POISON). The ø is prepared from dilution in alcohol. This poison produces muscular paralysis without impairing sensation or consciousness. Reflex action is diminished and a state of motor paralysis sets in. It decreases the output of adrenaline and brings about a state of nervous debility.

DROSERA. (SUNDEW). The ø is prepared from the fresh plant. The lymphatic and pleural systems together with synovial membranes are all affected by this plant. The laryngeal area is also subjected to inflammatory processes, any stimulus producing a hypersensitive reaction.

DULCAMARA. (WOODY NIGHTSHADE). The ø is prepared from the green stems and leaves before flowering. This plant belongs to the same family as Belladonna, Hyoscyamus and Stramonium: Tissue affinities are with mucous membranes, glands and kidneys, producing inflammatory changes and intestinal haemorrhages. This remedy may benefit those conditions which arise as a result of exposure to wet and cold, especially when damp evenings follow a warm day. Autumn diarrhoea should benefit.

ECHINACEA. (RUDBECKIA). The ø is prepared from the whole plant. Acute toxaemia with septic involvement of various tissues come within the sphere of action of this plant. It is a valuable remedy in the treatment of post-partum puerperal conditions where sepsis is evident. Generalised septic states having their origin in infected bites or stings will also benefit. This remedy acts best in low potencies.

FICUS RELIGIOSA. (PAKUR). The ø is prepared from fresh leaves in alcohol. Haemorrhages of various kinds are associated with the toxic effects of this plant. Any condition which produces bleeding of a bright red character may indicate the need for this remedy. It could be of value in coccidiosis but generally respiratory rather than digestive aspects determine its use.

GRANATUM. (POMEGRANATE). Potencies are prepared from the seeds. This is one of the remedies which is used in connection with round worm infestation.

GRAPHITES. Potencies are prepared from triturations dissolved in alcohol. This form of carbon has an affinity with skin and hooves. Eruptions are common and its action on connective tissue tends to produce fibrotic conditions associated with malnutrition. Loss of hair occurs while pimply moist eruptions ooze a sticky discharge. Abrasions develop into ulcers which may suppurate. Favourable sites for eczema are in the bends of joints and behind the ears.

GUNPOWDER. The ø is prepared from trituration and subsequent dilution in alcohol. This substance has proved its efficacy in the treatment of various conditions of a septic or toxic nature, e.g. abscesses, blood-poisoning and infected wounds.

HEPAR SULPHURIS CALCAREUM. This substance is prepared by burning crude calcium carbonate with flowers of sulphur. Potencies are then prepared from the triturated ash. This remedy is associated with suppurative processes producing conditions which are extremely sensitive to touch. It causes catarrhal and purulent inflammation of the mucous membranes of the respiratory and alimentary tracts with involvement of the skin and lymphatic system. This remedy has a wide range of action and should be considered in any suppurative process showing sensitivity to touch. Low potencies of this remedy promote suppuration while high potencies 200c and upwards may abort the purulent process and promote resolution.

HYDRASTIS CANADENSIS. (GOLDEN SEAL). The ø is prepared from the fresh root. Mucous membranes are affected by this plant, a catarrhal inflammation being established. Secretions generally are thick and yellow. Any catarrhal condition resulting in a muco–purulent discharge will come within the scope of this remedy, e.g. mild forms of metritis or sinusitis.

HYPERICUM PERFORATUM. (ST. JOHN'S WORT). The ø is prepared from the whole fresh plant. The main affinity is with the nervous system causing hypersensitivity, sloughing and necrosis of the skin may take place. This remedy is of prime importance in the treatment of lacerated wounds where nerve endings are damaged. In spinal injuries especially of the coccyx it gives good results. The specific action on nerves suggests its use in tetanus where, given early after injury, it helps prevent the spread of toxin. It can be used externally for lacerated wounds along with *CALENDULA* in a strength of 1/10.

IODUM. (IODINE. THE ELEMENT). Potencies are prepared from the tincture dissolved in alcohol. Iodine has a special affinity with the thyroid gland. Weakness and atrophy of muscles may follow excessive intake. The skin becomes dry and withered looking and appetite becomes voracious. It is a useful gland remedy in general.

IPECACUANHA. The ø is prepared from the dried root. Emetine alkaloid is its principal constituent. This plant is associated with haemorrhages and has found its use in practice in the treatment of post-partum bleeding where the blood comes in gushes, and in coccidiosis.

IRIS VERSICOLOR. (BLUE FLAG). The ø is prepared from the fresh root. This plant produces an action on various glands principally the salivary, pancreas and thyroid. The remedy is chiefly used in practice for treatment of pancreatic disorders where the stools become soft and creamy.

KALI BICHROMICUM. Potencies are prepared from a solution in distilled water. This salt acts on the mucous membranes of the stomach, intestines and respiratory tract with lesser involvement of other organs. Feverish states are absent. The action on the mucous membranes produces a catarrhal discharge of a tough stringy character of a yellow colour. This particular type of discharge is a strong guiding symptom for its use. It could be of use in broncho-pneumonia, sinusitis and pyelonephritis.

KALMIA LATIFOLIA. (MOUNTAIN LAUREL). The ø is prepared from fresh leaves. This plant has a prominent action on the heart. Large doses of the active principle reduces the general action considerably. The pulse becomes weak while palpitation is accompanied by fibrillation. It should be kept in mind as a remedy which could be of use in the cardiac form of Swine Erysipelas.

KAMALA. (CROTON COCCINEUS). Potencies are prepared from the powder obtained from the plant capsules and after trituration dissolved in alcohol. This is one of the main remedies to be considered in any worming programme especially tapeworm infestation.

KREOSOTUM. (CREOSOTE). The ø is prepared from solution in rectified spirit. This substance produces haemorrhages from small wounds with discharges and ulcerations. It also causes rapid decomposition of body fluids. Blepharitis occurs with a tendency to gangrene of the skin while in sows dark blood appears from the uterus. This substance has been successfully used in threatened gangrenous states showing the typical early stages of spongy ulceration and bleeding.

LACHESIS. (BUSHMASTER SNAKE). The ø is prepared from trituration of the venom dissolved in alcohol. This venom produces decomposition of blood rendering it more fluid.

There is a strong tendency to haemorrhage and sepsis with profound prostration. It is valuable if the throat develops inflammation causing left-sided swelling which may involve the parotid gland. Where haemorrhage takes place the blood is dark and does not clot readily while the skin surrounding any lesions assumes a purplish appearance. It could prove of value in the milder forms of Swine Erysipelis.

LATHYRUS SATIVUS. (CHICK PEA). The ø is prepared from the flower and the pods. This plant affects the anterior columns of the spinal cord producing paralysis of the lower extremities. Nerve power generally is weakened. It should be considered in recumbent conditions associated with mineral deficiencies and in any state involving nerve weakness leading to local paralysis.

LAURACERASUS. (CHERRY LAUREL). The ø is prepared from fresh young leaves. This shrub produces heart symptoms associated with coughing. Cyanosis develops and the skin feels cold. The valves are chiefly affected, mitral regurgitation being the chief pathological condition. This produces cyanosis with a small feeble pulse. This is one of the remedies which should be kept in mind when dealing with Swine Erysipelas.

LITHIUM CARBONICUM. (LITHIUM CARBONATE). The ø is prepared from trituration of the dried salt. This substance produces a chronic rheumatic-like state with a uric acid diathesis. It also has an action on the heart: Rheumatic-like stiffness and affections of joints especially carpal and metacarpal in the fore limbs and the hock and metatarsals in the hind.

LYCOPODIUM. (CLUB MOSS). The ø is prepared from the spores of the whole plant. The spores contain an active principle which acts chiefly on the renal and digestive systems. The respiratory system is also markedly affected. There is a general lack of gastric function and very little food is seen to satisfy the animal. The abdomen becomes bloated with tenderness over the liver. Stools are generally hard.

MAGNESIUM PHOSPHORICUM. Potencies are prepared from trituration of the salt in solution. This salt acts on muscles, producing a cramping effect with spasm. It is a valuable remedy to be remembered in supportive treatment in nervous conditions showing excessive stimulation of peripheral nerves.

MEDUSA. (JELLY FISH). Potencies are prepared from the whole animal, dissolved in alcohol. This substance has a marked action on the mammary glands producing milk in cases of agalactia. It should be remembered as a useful remedy in agalactia in the sow and could profitably be combined with *E. coli* in specific conditions.

MERCURIUS CORROSIVUS. (MERCURIC CHLORIDE). Potencies are prepared from triturations and subsequent dilution. This salt produces severe straining of the lower bowel leading to dysentery and also has a destructive action on the kidneys. Discharges from mucous surfaces assume a greenish tinge. It could be of value in severe cases of occidiosis.

MEZEREUM. (SPURGE OLIVE). The ø is prepared from fresh bark. The active principle of this plant produces symptoms of skin involvement together with intestinal affections.

Eczema occurs with severe itching. Vesicles arise which progress to ulcer formation in a surrounding red area. When scabs form they tend to become under-run with pus. It could be of value in skin conditions such as mange.

MILLEFOLIUM. (YARROW). The ø is prepared from the whole fresh plant. This plant produces haemorrhages from various parts, the blood being bright red. Nasal bleeding occurs with bleeding from the lungs. Haemorrhages occur from the bowels and also from the urinary tract. Sows may show bright red blood post partum.

NATRUM MURIATICUM. (COMMON SALT). Potencies are prepared from triturations dissolved in distilled water. Excessive intake of salt leads to anaemia evidenced by oedema of various parts. White blood cells are increased while mucous membranes are rendered dry. This is a remedy which is of value in unthrifty conditions arising as a result of chronic nephritis.

NUX VOMICA. (POISON NUT). The ø is prepared from the seeds. Digestive disturbances and congestions are associated with this plant, flatulence and indigestion being commonly encountered. Stools are generally hard.

PALLADIUM. (THE METAL). Potencies are prepared from trituration and subsequent dilution in alcohol. This element produces its main action on the female genital system especially the ovaries causing an inflammation with a tendency to pelvic peritonitis. The right ovary is more usually affected. Pelvic disorders arising as a result of ovaritis should benefit.

PAREIRA. (VELVET LEAF). The ø is prepared from tincture of fresh root. The active principle of this plant exerts its action mainly on the urinary system producing catarrhal inflammation of the bladder with a tendency to stone formation. In the sow there may be vaginal or uterine discharge. It is a useful remedy to consider in cases of vesical calculus where the animal is presented with acute straining and distress.

PETROLEUM. (ROCK SPIRIT). The ø is prepared from the oil. This substance produces cutaneous eruptions and catarrh from muscous membranes. Eczematous eruptions develop around ears and eyelids and feet producing fissures which are slow to heal. The skin is usually dry. Complaints are usually worse in cold weather. A useful remedy for some forms of chronic skin conditions where symptoms agree.

PHOSPHORUS. (THE ELEMENT). The ø is prepared from trituration of red phosphorus. This important substance produces an inflammatory and degenerative effect on mucous membranes, and causes bone destruction and necrosis of the liver and other organs. It has a profound effect on eye structures especially the retina and iris. There is a marked haemorrhagic tendency associated with this remedy: small haemorrhages appear on the skin and mucous membranes. Its use in practice is wide and varied.

PHYTOLOCCA DECANDRA. (POKE ROOT). The ø is prepared from the whole fresh plant. A state of restlessness and prostration is associated with this plant, together with glandular swellings. It is chiefly used to combat swellings of the mammary glands in particular when the glands become hard and painful. Abscesses may develop together with mastitis of varying degree. In the male testicular swelling may occur. The remedy is of immense value in mastitis and other forms of mammary swellings.

PITUITARY. The ø is prepared from the whole gland. The remedy is used as a help in conditions where there is an imbalance in the animals hormonal system. It can be combined with any other hormonal remedy to enhance the action.

PLATINA. (THE METAL PLATINUM). The ø is prepared from trituration of the metal with lactose and subsequent dilution in alcohol. This metal has a specific action on the female genital system especially the ovaries where inflammation readily develops. Cystic ovaries develop frequently.

PODOPHYLLUM. (MAY APPLE). The ø is prepared from the whole fresh plant. The active principle of this plant exerts its action mainly on the small intestine causing an enteritis. The liver and rectum are also affected. Distension of the abdomen occurs with a tendency to lie on the abdomen. A watery greenish diarrhoea may alternate with constipation. It is a useful remedy to remember in the context of the many enteric conditions which can affect young pigs.

PLUMBUM METALLICUM. (THE METAL LEAD). The ø is prepared from trituration with sugar of milk dissolved in alcohol. A state of paralysis preceded by pain is produced by exposure to or ingestion of lead. It affects the central nervous system and also causes liver damage leading to jaundice. Anaemia develops. Paralysis of lower limbs develops and convulsions are common leading to coma.

PSORIUNUM. SCABIES VESICLE. The ø is prepared from trituration of the dried vesicle. This nosode produces a state of debility especially after illness with skin symptoms predominating. All discharges are unpleasant. Skin conditions are accompanied by severe itching. Animals needing this remedy prefer warmth.

PULSATILLA. (ANEMONE). The ø is prepared from the entire plant when in flower. Mucous membranes come within the sphere of action of this plant, thick muco-purulent discharges being produced. It has proved useful in the treatment of ovarian hypofunction and in retained placenta.

PYROGEN. (ARTIFICIAL SEPSIN). The ø is prepared from solution of raw protein in distilled water. This nosode has a specific relation to septic inflammations associated with offensive discharges. It is indicated in all septic conditions where the animal presents a clinical picture of raised temperature alternating with a weak thready pulse or vice versa. It should be used in potencies of 200c and upwards.

RHUS TOXICODENDRON. (POISON IVY). The ø is prepared from the fresh leaves. The active principles of this tree affect skin and muscles together with mucous membranes and fibrous tissues producing blistery eruptions. Symptoms of stiffness are relieved by movement, a reddish rash develops on the skin with vesicles. This remedy could prove useful in the chronic form of Swine Erysipelas and also in some skin conditions of an allergic origin.

RUTA GRAVEOLENS. (RUE). The ø is prepared from the whole fresh plant. Ruta produces its action on the periosteum and cartilages with a secondary action on eyes and uterus. Deposits form particularly around the carpal joints. It also has a selective action on the lower bowel and rectum.

SABINA. (SAVINE). The ø is prepared from the oil dissolved in alcohol. The uterus is the main seat of action producing a tendency to abortion. It is associated with haemorrhages of bright red blood which remains fluid. This remedy has its main use in uterine conditions including retained placenta.

It could prove a useful remedy along with *CAULOPHYLLUM* in helping to prevent abortions in various diseases where this could be a hazard, e.g. Respiratory and Reproductive Disease.

SAMBUCUS NIGRA. (ELDER). The ø is prepared from fresh leaves and flowers. The action of the active principle of this tree is chiefly on the respiratory system. Accumulation of mucus in the larynx may impede normal respiration. Coughing develops. This remedy should be remembered along with other relevant ones in the many conditions which affect the respiratory system of growing pigs.

SECALE CORNUTUM. (ERGOT OF RYE). The ø is prepared from the fresh fungus. Ergot produces marked contraction of smooth muscle causing a diminution of blood supply to various areas This is particularly seen in peripheral blood vessels especially of the feet. Stools are dark green, sometimes dysenteric. Bleeding of dark blood occurs from the uterus with putrid discharges. This remedy could prove useful in conditions such as Vibrionic Dysentery and Swine Erysipelas.

SELENIUM. (THE ELEMENT). The ø is prepared from trituration with lactose and dilution in alcohol or distilled water. The skin and the genito-urinary systems are involved with this remedy. Weakness of bladder muscle leads to a loss of power to expel urine. Dryness and itching of skin develops especially around the feet. Alopecia and eruptions are also seen.

SEPIA. (INK OF CUTTLE FISH). Potencies are prepared from trituration of the dried liquid. Disturbances of the female genital system are associated with this remedy. Prolapse of the uterus may occur. It will regulate the entire oestrus cycle and should always be given as a routine preliminary remedy in treatment. It also acts on the skin producing roughened whitish areas. Post-partum discharges of various sorts will usually respond. It is also useful in encouraging the maternal instinct of sows which may be indifferent to their young.

SILICEA. (PURE FLINT). Potencies are prepared from trituration dissolved in alcohol. The main action of this substance is on bone where it is capable of causing caries and necrosis. It also causes abscesses and fistulae of connective tissue with secondary fibrous growths. There is a tendency for all wounds to suppurate. This is a widely used remedy indicated in many suppurative processes of a chronic nature. It should prove useful in promoting healthy growth of horn in boars especially which develop weak hooves.

SPONGIA. (ROASTED SPONGE). Potencies are prepared from dilutions in alcohol. This substance has an action on the respiratory and cardiac systems. The thyroid gland becomes enlarged. It is generally used as a heart remedy after respiratory infections. It could be helpful in heart complications of Swine Erysipelas.

STAPHISAGRIA. (STAVESACRE). The ø is prepared from the seeds. This remedy is not often called for in pig practice but it could prove useful in some forms of cystitis but more importantly as a post-operative remedy which aids healing after surgical interference.

STRAMONIUM. (THORN APPLE). The ø is prepared from the whole fresh plant and fruit. The active principle of this shrub produces its main action on the central nervous system especially the cerebrum producing a staggering gait with a tendency to fall on the left side. Dilation of the pupils occurs with a fixed staring look. This remedy should be considered in disturbances of the central nervous system showing typical symptoms.

STRYCHNINUM. (STRYCHNINE). Potencies are prepared from solution in water. With this remedy all reflexes are rendered more active and pupils become dilated. Rigidity of muscles occurs especially of the neck and back with jerking and twitching of limbs. Muscle tremors and tetanic convulsions set in rapidly. Various cerebrospinal affections may be helped by this remedy.

SULPHUR. (THE ELEMENT). Potencies are prepared from trituration and subsequent dilution in alcohol. This remedy has a wide range of action but is chiefly used in skin conditions such as mange and eczema.

SYMPHYTUM. (COMFREY). The ø is prepared from the fresh plant. The root of this plant produces a substance which stimulates the growth of epithelium on ulcerated surfaces and hastens the union of bone in fractures. It has a limited use in pig practice.

TARENTULA CUBENSIS. (CUBAN SPIDER). The ø is prepared from trituration of the whole insect. The poison of this spider produces a toxic condition with septic complications. Papular reddish eruptions develop on the skin together with carbuncles and boils. The skin assumes a purplish appearance.

TEREBINTHINAE. (OIL OF TURPENTINE). Potencies are prepared from a solution in alcohol. Haemorrhages are prepared from various surfaces, urinary symptoms predominating.

There is difficulty in urinating. Post-partum haemorrhages may develop. It is chiefly used in acute kidney conditions associated with haematuria and a sweet-smelling urine, which has been likened to violets.

TEUCRIUM MARUM. (CAT THYME). The ø is prepared from the whole fresh plant. Although this plant has an action on both the respiratory and alimentary systems it should be chiefly remembered as a homoeopathic worming remedy and can be used in alternation with others such as *KAMALA* and *GRANATUM*.

THALLIUM ACETAS. (THALLIUM ACETATE). Potencies are prepared by trituration of the salt dissolved in alcohol. This metal exerts an action on the endocrine system and also on the skin and neuro-muscular system where it produces paralysis followed by muscular atrophy. Skin conditions frequently result in alopecia. It is used mainly in the treatment of trophic skin conditions such as alopecia and myelitis.

TRILLIUM PENDULUM. (WHITE BETH-ROOT). The ø is prepared from the fresh root. Haemorrhages are produced along with blood-stained mucous diarrhoea. Bleeding of bright red blood takes place from the uterus. It should be remembered as a useful remedy in uterine bleeding especially if this is associated with alimentary symptoms of loose stools.

TUBERCULINUM AVIARE. This is the nosode of avian tuberculosis and is used in pig practice as a remedy to aid convalescence after influenza and bronchitis.

URTICA URENS. (STINGING NETTLE). The ø is prepared from the fresh plant. This plant causes loss of milk with a tendency to the formation of calculi in the urine. Urticarial swellings develop on the skin. Urine output is diminished. The mammary glands become enlarged with surrounding oedema. This is a very useful remedy in various renal and skin conditions and also in agalactia where high potencies will help promote milk.

USTILLAGO MAYDIS. (CORN SMUT). The ø is prepared from trituration of the fungus and dilution in alcohol. This substance has an affinity with the genital organs of both sexes particularly sows and gilts where the uterus is markedly affected. Haemorrhages occur post-partum.

UVA URSI. (BEARBERRY). The ø is prepared from dried leaves and fruit. The active principle of this plant is associated with disturbances of the urinary system. Cystitis occurs, the urine containing blood, pus and mucus. Purulent inflammation is confined to the kidney pelvis. This is one of the main remedies to consider in the treatment of cystitis and pyelonephritis.

VARIOLINUM. This is the nosode of smallpox and potencies are prepared from the virus dissolved in alcohol. It should be remembered as a useful remedy in the treatment of Swine Pox. In any outbreak of this disease all in-contact animals should be protected by this nosode.

VERATRUM ALBUM. (WHITE HELLEBORE). The ø is prepared from root stocks. A picture of collapse is presented by the action of this plant. Extremities become cold and signs of cyanosis appear. Purging occurs, the watery stools being accompanied by exhaustion. The body becomes cold and stools are greenish. Signs of abdominal pain precede the onset of diarrhoea.

VIBURNUM OPULIS. (WATER ELDER). The ø is prepared from the fresh bark. The female genital system is markedly affected, chiefly the uterus, producing a tendency to abortion in the first quarter of pregnancy, sterility being a common sequel. It should be given as a routine in breeding herds.

INDEX

*W*HEN USING THE index, please begin with the specific (e.g. coughing) and work back to the general (e.g. respiratory problems). Entries use the words shown in the text and there are consequently several ways of describing a condition (e.g. apathy, depression, lethargy etc): although cross references to similar and related terms are given, if you cannot find the particular word you would use to describe the condition please look up a similar term which should lead to the information you need.